In Her Own Words...

VIRGINIA SATIR
Selected Papers 1963 - 1983

Edited by John Banmen

ZEIG, TUCKER & THEISEN, INC.

Phoenix   Arizona

Published by

ZEIG, TUCKER & THEISEN, INC.
3618 North 24th Street
Phoenix, AZ 85016

Manufactured in the United States of America

In Her Own Words

Contents

Contributors

Dr. Pindy Badyal, Ph.D., psychologist, AAMFT approved supervisor

Sharon Blevins, M.S., GC-C, teacher, counselor, trainer

Dr. Jesse Carlock, Ph.D., psychologist, associate editor, *Satir Journal*

Moira Haagen, M.Ed., individual and family therapy

Colleen Murphy, M.Ed., instructor Douglas College, family therapist

Sandy Novak, M.Ed., M.A., Adjunct Senior Faculty, Naropa University

Dr. Stuart Piddocke, M.A., Ph.D., retired anthropology professor

Dr. Carl Sayles, Psy.D., LMFT, marriage and family therapist

Stephen Smith, M.S.W., addiction counsellor and family therapist

Gloria Taylor, M.A., Adjunct professor, Waterloo Lutheran Seminary

Introduction   by John Banmen

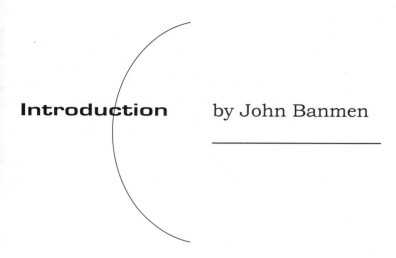

I attended my first workshop with Virginia Satir one month after I completed my graduate studies. My studies in counseling psychology used a very structured Rogerian model that allowed and even encouraged the clients to free associate their thoughts and feelings with the therapist, practicing genuine acceptance and empathy. One of the first clinical observations I made was of Virginia Satir's constantly asking questions while working with the participants of the group. It felt like Socrates incarnate. At that time I did not realize that the questions were generally focused and positively directional at the experiential level. I was more impressed by her magic, than by her skills and understanding her approach. Looking back now, that five-day residential workshop changed me and my therapeutic practice forever. Two years later I had the chance to spend three months with her as she worked with the Manitoba, Canada government, health organizations, health professionals and the public.

Virginia Satir was born in 1916 and lived until September of 1988. She was born in Wisconsin on a farm. Her parents were Christian Scientists of German descent. She was the oldest of five children. Bright, competent and very curious about life and learning, she entered Milwaukee State Teachers College at the age of sixteen. She graduated in 1936, with a Bachelor of Education degree, before turning 20 years old. She had numerous teaching jobs until 1941 when she enrolled at the School of Social Work at the University of Chicago. After graduating with a master's degree in social work and after working for some time at the Chicago Home for Girls, she opened a private practice. She conducted her first family session in 1951 (Brothers, 2000).

Satir worked at the Illinois State Psychiatric Institute until 1958 when she moved to California. It wasn't long until she joined Don Jackson to help start the Mental Research Institute. She is considered one of the founders of MRI, which continues to be a major institution in the family therapy movement. Eventually, she moved to Esalen as director of training. By 1968 she left Esalen to spend full time offering workshops around the world. (For a detailed biographical sketch see Brothers, 2000.)

Virgin Satir is internationally recognized for her creativity as one of the co-founders of family therapy. Based on the conviction that people are capable of continued growth, change, and new understanding, her goal was to improve relationships and communication within the family. She once said that in healing the family we heal the world. In her early years at the Mental Research Institute, her model was often associated with the communication based approach for understanding and interpreting family dysfunction. Unfortunately, this label is clearly a misnomer for the highly transformational systemic therapeutic approach that she developed in the last decade of her life. By the mid1960s, Satir had already expanded the communications approach of her communication stances to include affective, mind-body and spiritual domains.

Satir, the founder of what more recently has been called the Satir Transformational Systemic Therapy, saw counseling/therapy as an intense experience with the inner self. Because she was more a teacher and trainer than a writer she did not publish as much as some of her contemporaries. Therefore, we are fortunate to be able to bring some of her unpublished manuscripts to the current helping profession as well as to re-issue some of her published material. We have undertaken this project not just to honor her contributions, but more important to utilize her wisdom, her insights, and her world-view in helping us in our present professional attempts to help others.

Virginia Satir is well recognized as one of the co-founders of family therapy alongside Murray Bowen, Nathan Ackerman and Carl Whitaker. Sal Minuchin and others joined the founding leaders at a slightly later date. A recent major research study (*Psychotherapy Networker*, March 2007) found that Satir ranked fifth on the list of the most influential therapists of the last 25 years. Her 1964 book called *Conjoint Family Therapy* challenged the prevailing practice of that time of seeing only individuals rather than whole families. Working very much in isolation from other family therapists at the beginning of her therapeutic career, she developed a style and form that was based on her own experience, her own beliefs, and her own intuitive capacity to see deeper into the core or essence of human yearnings. She saw her clients as loving, caring, struggling, hurting people who had the innate capacity and resources to learn and then to change their way of coping into a more responsible, empowered way of life.

Some of the basic tenants of her growth model of transformation are briefly noted here to help the reader to anchor her writings more succinctly.

1. We are basically positively directionally driven by our unique manifestation of the universal life force.

2. We have the internal resources to move beyond the basic coping level as well as the ability to harness our external resources in order to grow.

3. We can change the impact of earlier and present negative life experiences although we need not, and sometimes cannot, change the events and circumstances.

4. Therapy can and must operate at a deeper than the symptom level. Therapy often must work at the level of self to bring about healing and transformation.

5. The family system is the basic learning and living unit and, as such, needs to be included directly or indirectly in all therapy.

6. Change is always possible, at least internally where change usually needs to begin even when working with couples and families.

7. Making deep contact with the person and then creating an open, trusting, accepting relationship is a necessary component of therapy.

8. People are basically good, but sometimes need help to experience and manifest this aspect of themselves.

9. Feelings belong to people and therefore can be managed and often transformed into positive energy.

10. The use of the self of the therapist is an important ingredient of therapy. This means that the therapist has to evolve to a higher level of congruence and be able to tap into the life energy that connects the therapist and the client(s) during the therapeutic process.

11. The problem is not the problem, coping is. This conceptualization helps therapy to deal better with the underlying issues below the symptoms. It stresses the *being* more than the *doing*.

12. Therapy needs to focus on health and possibilities instead of pathology – not just what was and is, but what can become – to be more fully human.

13. Hope is a necessary component or ingredient for change to take place.

14. People connect on the basis of sameness and then grow through their differences.

These and hopefully other tenants of the Satir Transformational System Therapy model will become clearer as you read the various chapters of the book.

Satir advocated at least four basic, universal or meta-goals for all her therapy. In brief they focus on the following areas:

1. **Responsibility**: Clients would be helped to become more responsible for their actions, feelings, thoughts, expectations and to become more capable to meet their yearnings.

2. **Better Choice Makers**: With greater awareness and acceptance of themselves and perhaps with greater self-love, clients would learn to make better, meaning healthier, more wholesome choices in the context of self and others -- intrapsychically and interactively. Choices would be relational in terms of self, other, and situation.

3. **Self-Esteem**: Clients would be helped to raise their self-esteem. Self-esteem, as defined by Satir, meant how positively

people experience themselves and their life at the level of essence, not just how good they feel. Striving only to feel good could lead to narcissistic patterns of self-aggrandizing. Self-esteem is a state of *being* that includes congruence with the self, not just with one's feelings.

4. **Congruence**: Congruence is a state of harmony with one's inner self. It is being in tune with one's life energy. It is a connectedness with the universal, with all living human beings and beyond. Others might have called it self-actualizing or living in the Now. Satir called it peace within, peace between, and peace among.

With these four meta-goals for all clients, the therapist and client(s) can focus on individual and family goals in terms of their person-specific struggles and yearnings. Her month-long training programs during the 1970s and her month-long Process Communities of the 1980s were primarily focused on these four universal goals.

When people think of Virginia Satir, they often remember her as a teacher of coping stances: placating, blaming, computing, and irrelevant in sculpting format. In her book *New People Making* (Satir, 1988) she explained these thoroughly. Instead of limiting these by seeing them as merely "communication patterns," we should look at them as signs of where clients live in their *iceberg* in their survival state and use them to make contact with clients..

To convey her thoughts, her intentions, her view, her process, Satir would often use metaphors. Her most frequently used metaphor was that of sculpting—externalizing the internal and sculpting dysfunctional relationships using her coping stances. Another metaphor she often used in her therapeutic process was the iceberg metaphor.

The "iceberg" refers to a person, and so it includes a person's behavior, feelings, feelings about feelings, perceptions (cognition and beliefs), expectations and yearning, all sitting on the core, which is the Self, the "I AM." In the iceberg metaphor, Satir includes both spirit and soul. Soul is the seat of the mental and emotional complex that makes up our inner life. It is the translation of the Greek work *psyche*. Spirit, by contrast, is pure consciousness, the Self, the true "I AM."

Figure 1: The Personal Iceberg Metaphor

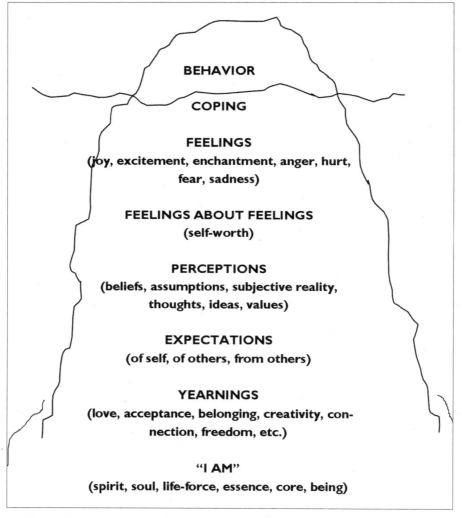

Satir, V., Banmen, J., Gerber, J. and Gomori, M. (1991)
The Satir Model: family therapy and beyond

Various therapeutic schools place more emphasis on one aspect of the iceberg over another aspect. Satir aimed to be inclusive and integrative. The iceberg metaphor gave her a way to include the basic psychological and spiritual processed that needed to be included in her form of transformational, systemic therapy.

Over time, Satir developed numerous therapeutic tools. In particular, she developed family reconstruction. It is an experiential means of helping individuals resolve unfinished business of one's childhood, reclaim ones resources or strengths and establish a healthy relationship with parents at the level of personhood. Much has been written about these processes (Wegscheider-Cruse, 1980, Nerin, 1986, 1993, Satir, Banmen, Gerber and Gomori, 1991, Banmen, 2006, Banmen, 2008).

Satir also developed a powerful tool called "parts-party" that helps integrate and empower the individual to achieve some greater degree of wholeness and congruence. This has now been developed so it can be used with one individual in an office setting, (Satir, et al, 1991). This has now been developed in an office setting (Maki-Banmen, 200?).

Moving from the external communication patterns to an internal communication pattern, Satir developed the internal *ingredience of an interaction* (Satir et al, 1991) to help therapists and clients track and intervene at various internal stages of processing one's experience.

Satir's five basic essential therapeutic elements are briefly described as follows:

1. *Experiential.* The therapy must be experiential, which means that the client is experiencing the impact of a past event in the present. At the same time, the client is experiencing his/ her own positive Life Energy in the present. Often, body memory is accessed as one of the ways to help clients experience impacts. It is only when clients are experiencing both the negative energy of the impact and the positive energy of their Life Force in the now that an energetic shift can take place.

2. *Systemic.* Therapy must work within the intrapsychic and interactive systems in which the client experiences his/her life. The intrapsychic system includes the emotions, perceptions, expectations, yearnings, and spiritual energy of the individual, all of which interact with each other in a systemic manner. The interactive systems include the relationships, both past and present, that the person has experienced. The two systems interact with each other. A change in one impacts the other. However, transformational change is an en-

ergetic shift in the intrapsychic system which that changes the interactive systems.

3. *Positively directional.* In the Satir Growth Model, the therapist actively engages with the client to help reframe perceptions, generate possibilities, hear the positive message of universal yearnings, and connect the client to his/her positive Life Energy. The focus is on health and possibilities, appreciating resources, and anticipating growth rather than on pathologizing or problem solving.

4. *Change focused.* As the focus of Satir therapy is on transformational change, the process questions asked throughout the entire therapy session are change related. Questions such as, "What would have to change for you to forgive yourself?" give the client an opportunity to explore uncharted waters inside of his/her own intrapsychic system.

5. *Self of the therapist.* As previously mentioned, the congruence of the therapist is essential for clients to access their own spiritual Life Energy. When therapists are congruent, clients experience them as caring, accepting, hopeful, interested, genuine, authentic, and actively engaged. Therapists' use of their own creative Life Energy in the form of metaphor, humor, self-disclosure, sculpting, and many other creative interventions also comes from the connection that therapists have to their own spiritual Self when in a congruent state.

The eleven chapters of this book are produced in chronological order from 1963 to 1983. Some have been published in books while others have never been published.

I have a writers group of therapists trained in the Satir Model who meet regularly to encourage each other to write, provide feedback, and do some projects such as producing some video tapes for educational purposes. Group members collected all the published and unpublished articles and chapters they could find with the help of the Virginia Satir archives at the University of California, Santa Barbara where Carl Rogers archives are also kept.

We had over thirty chapters and articles published and unpublished and selected the enclosed eleven for inclusion in this book. Several articles seemed like different versions of the same material. Several had much overlapping material and some were in their early draft form. We selected what the group considered the best. Each member then took one chapter and produced the introduction to it. One person produced the introduction to two chapters. Each member of the group participated in each others editing of "their" chapter. The chapters are presented in chronological order to give readers a flavor of Satir's intellectual journey. Each chapter has a short introduction written by a contemporary practitioner who offers a few words of context and focus for what follows.

Finally, as the chapters are taken from live presentations, unpublished written material and earlier published articles, a prudent amount of editing was done in effort to clarify important information without interfering with her lively communication style.

In the first chapter of this book, *Schizophrenia and Family Therapy,* first published in 1963, Virginia Satir sees and advocated the need to work with the whole family and look at the symptom as a form of action and reaction that can be resolved through systemic intervention.

In chapter two, *The Family as a Treatment Unit,* Satir gives the reader a sense of open and closed family systems and how restrictive communication rules often hamper the health of individuals and families and what can be done about it.

In chapter three, *Family Systems and Approaches to Family Therapy,* Satir looks back at some therapeutic history and shares her work at the *Mental Research Institute* regarding family systems thinking. Her comments might be the forerunner of the internal process of individuals while communicating with others. It later became know as the *ingredients of an interaction* (Satir et al., 1991).

In chapter four, *The Growing Edge of Myself as a Family Therapist,* Satir describes her move from the prevailing psychoanalytical approach of the day to working with her first family by violating some "cardinal rules". She developed at that time the use of chronological history that gave families a reliable way to place the family in time and context (Satir et al, 1991). She also mentions some of her major interventions that soon followed.

In chapter five, *Making a One-Parent Family Work,* Satir describes how to create a wholesome environment by a single parent and how to meet the needs of the children, including their spiritual needs while adjusting to the new family situation. With the divorce rate much higher now than 30 years ago, this chapter is a very helpful guide for present practicing therapists.

In chapter six, *Conjoint Family Therapy,* Satir again talks about working within the family system, changing the system instead of *correcting* the symptom. Through an experiential approach of raising one's self-esteem, family members will accept them selves and each other and develop an open, supportive, hopeful relationship. Satir describes what healthy families look like and what part the therapist plays in promoting family members to change through process rather than behavioral outcomes.

In chapter seven, *A Partial Portrait of a Family Therapist in Progress,* Satir provides us some of her early history and experiences of developing her own approach and how she met other family therapy founders along the way. She describes her eight different levels of health through the use of the *Mandala* (Buckbee, 2007) emphasizing her health oriented approach in therapy.

In chapter eight, *The Therapist and Family Therapy,* Satir writes about her belief that all humans can grow, that we have the resources to change, that symptoms signal blockages in the flow of life energy that actually provide a (dysfunctional) survival purpose. The whole chapter is written in a historical developmental context describing many of her approaches and interventions and beliefs she uses in therapy. She include an initial interview to demonstrate her beliefs and approach.

In chapter nine, *When I Meet a Person,* Satir reflects on her experience she recently had with a family. She covers many of her beliefs, her style, her approach and her won internal experience while doing therapy. She explains her use of the client's energy field very much like energy medicine (Orloff, 2004) and energy psychology (Feinstein et al., 2005) do today.

In chapter ten, *Therapist's Use of Self,* Satir emphasizes the need of the therapist to be congruent (Banmen, 2007) to the point of connecting from the level of the Self (see iceberg metaphor described earlier) with the level of yearning of the client and using the life energy of both to achieve some transformational change. The use of self has become an important topic in the therapeutic literature (Balwin, M. (ed.), 2000).

In chapter eleven, *The Therapist Story,* Satir continues her emphasis on the use of self of the therapist in building a healing relationship with the family and family members and how the use of self can and needs to be of a positive value in therapy.

It is my privilege and honor to help bring these writings of Virginia Satir to the professional public, some articles for the first time. It is now twenty years since her death. Her words, her insights, her messages seem very helpful, relevant and inspiring in the 21st century. Now, without further explication from me, I invite you, the reader to enjoy the wisdom of Virginia Satir *In Her Own Words.*

— John Banmen, Editor
January 2008

References

Baldwin, M. ed., (2000). *The use of self in therapy.* 2nd Ed. New York, NY. Haworth Press.

Banmen, J. ed., (2006). *Applications of the Satir growth model.* Seattle, WA: Avanta: The Virginia Satir Network.

Banmen, J. ed., (2007). *Satir transformational systemic therapy.* Palo Alto, CA: Science and Behavior books, Inc.

Brothers, B. J. Virginia Satir. In Suhd, M., Dodson, L., Gomori, M., ed. (2000). *Virginia Satir: Her life and circle of influence.* Palo Alto, CA: Science and Behavior Books, Inc.

Buckbee, S. An overview of the Satir mandala. In Banmen, J. (ed), (2006). *Applications of the Satir growth model.* Seattle, WA. Avanta: The Virginia Satir Network.

Feinstein, D., Eden, D. and Graig, G. (2005). *The promise of energy psychology.* New York, NY: Jeremy P. Tarcher/Penguin.

Nerin, E. F. (1986). *Family Reconstruction: Long days journey into light.* New York, NY: Norton and Company.

Nerin, W. F. (1993). *You can't grow up till you go back home.* New York, NY: Crossroad.

Orloff, J. (2004). *Positive Energy.* New York, NY: Harmony Books.

Satir, V., Banmen, J., Gerber, J., Gomori, M. (1991). *The Satir model: Family therapy and beyond.* Palo Alto, CA: Science and Behavior Books, Inc.

Wegscheider–Cruse, S., Higby, K., Klontz, T., and Rainey, A. (1994) *Family reconstruction: A living theater model.* Palo Alto, CA: Science and Behavior Books, Inc.

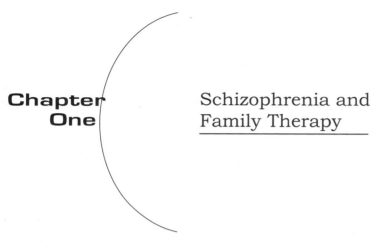

Chapter One

Schizophrenia and Family Therapy

Introduction by Sandy Novak

Deceptively simple! That's how Satir's work has often been described. Yet those who have delved into her model have found it to be profound in its simplicity.

Satir presents her central and, perhaps, greatest contributions, in this article. She breaks from traditional psychology (Freud's drive theory) and introduces her seminal view that the way we develop a sense of self is through the "blueprint" our family gives us about how to see the world, ourselves, and ourselves in relationships. On this insight she will build her transformational therapy, for if we are to break free of the dysfunctional elements in the original blueprint, then we need to transform these internalized lessons.

Another of her brilliant insights into the nature of human beings is her observation of the impact of incongruence in the family on a developing child. The research in the 1950s by Gregory Bateson and his group asserted that schizophrenia was caused by "double binds" put on the child by the incongruent messages of one parent. Satir noted that parents often have differences of opinion or style, and a problem develops if they will not acknowledge those differences. Somehow the child has to unify his experience and make sense of incongruities. In this article, Satir advances an alternative to the theory proposed by the Bateson group. She observed that the two parents are bound by rules that do not permit them to openly criticize each other or even disagree with each other. In cre-

ating the impression that they are duplicates, they cause sy
matic behavior in children. Since no two people are exactl
the child senses the unspoken differences and will act out tru
"delusion."

Her paper is rich with helpful descriptors of components of
healthy, functional families where differences can be questioned,
confronted, and honored. Long before stress became a buzzword,
she defines it systemically for us.

She challenges the family therapist to work on her own congru-
ity, a theme she develops throughout her later works around the
use of the self of the therapist.

■ ■ ■

Family therapy is a new approach to problems familiar to all
who work in the field of mental health. I define it as a method by
which all persons currently in a family, in which there is an
identified patient with a symptom, are asked to come together at
the same time and in the same place.

The theory that the patient should be seen in the context of
his total family is based upon the premise that the patient's
symptom is as much a manifestation of his interpretation of the
action, interaction, and reaction of his parents as it is a manifestation of him. When I use the word *parents* I am always thinking
of three simultaneous relationships: male and female; husband
and wife; and mother and father. Seeing the family together
makes it possible to understand the network of actions and reactions of everyone in the family, and the symptom is seen as one
form of action and reactions.

The *schizophrenic family*, that is, a family in which there is an
individual clinically labeled as a schizophrenic, can be described
in a general way as one in which the parents of the schizophrenic child (who may, of course, be over twenty-one) behave as
though they are strictly bound by rules that do not permit them
openly and directly to criticize each other, or to disagree with
each other about each other. Thus they create the impression
that they are duplicates. Their differentness cannot be acknowledged, and their unspoken criticisms and disagreements are reflected in a caricatured and thinly disguised way in their child's
behavior.

No two people are exactly the same, and if the husband and
wife keep up the illusion, with each other, with their child, and

with the outside world, that they do not have disagreements, that they are not different from each other, and that they do not have critical feelings toward each other, their delusion will be reflected in the child's behavior. The parent's picture of supposed perfection, implying exact similarity, says to the child, "Be like me. Be without anger. Do not disagree." To attempt to do this is incompatible with reality, growth, and the development of individuality and sexuality. The patient instead has to develop a pattern of behavior that can accommodate: "I am growing; I am not growing. It is real; it is not real. I am an individual; I am not an individual."

In the context of family therapy, schizophrenia is considered one of several symptoms that indicate family dysfunction. Like other symptoms, it is a comment on the person—a sign that his growth has been distorted—while at the same time it is an SOS, giving clues to the presence of pain or trouble in those persons who have survival significance for the child, such as parents. If we consider schizophrenia a symptom, then "schizophrenia" also becomes a descriptive term that labels an individual's behavior as strange to those who observe him and interact with him. Other symptoms, in other contexts, carry the messages that a person's behavior is sick (psychosomatic illness), stupid (mentally retarded, underachieving), or bad (delinquent, criminal, alcoholic, narcotic). Family interaction will be different as symptoms differ.

Concepts of individual psychotherapy usually point to an etiology of symptomatology within the individual who has the symptom. In contrast, as a practitioner of family therapy, I see a symptom as an outcome of a family learning system that involves parents and their children, for whom they are survival figures. The parents will be the models from whom the developing infant learns his blueprint. The blueprint evolves from concepts that the child forms about labeling (what he calls things, people, and ideas), and from the meaning he attaches to those labels, a process I call *coding*. He learns to label and code both himself and others, both in his private world and in the outside world.

Each individual is unique, even though some people try to deny it. Inevitably, each parent looks different, sounds different, and has different ideas, all of which the child must integrate into his blueprint. The ease with which he is able to do this will depend upon the techniques his parents have worked out for recognizing their differences, for explicitly labeling them, and for integrating them in order to achieve jointly desired outcomes.

I should add, parenthetically, that all families have to deal with a paradox of learning. The child does not know that the parents do not know that the child does not understand why they do what they do. The child acts as though the parents see and know him as he knows and sees himself. The parents act as though the child knows them and sees them as they see themselves. These illusions are not discovered until either the child or a parent behaves in some unexpected way. Yet this surprising behavior occurs because the child acts consistently with his level of growth, and the parent acts consistently with the fact that adults have many habitual automatic responses that the child has not learned to understand. This dilemma of "not knowing" can become another positive means of learning by which the child develops his blueprint, but only if parent and child are able to be explicit with each other.

A child develops his blueprint by what he hears his parents say—separately and together—or to others in his presence; by what they tell him directly—separately and together in his presence—and by what they permit him to do—separately and together in his presence. The child will seek to unify his experiences in these situations; and so far in our studies with families we have outlined five general ways in which he does this. A child may reject his mother's way and accept his father's way; conversely, he may reject the father's way and accept the mother's way. A third possibility is that he will reject both mother and father and will choose as a model a grandmother, an older sister or brother, or some person outside the family, such as a teacher or a probation officer. In functioning families the child takes what fits him from both his mother and father. The schizophrenic solution is to choose neither mother nor father, and to behave as if they are both the same, thus trying to fit the illusion of sameness presented by the parents to the child as reality. This idea of reality, reflected by the child, is delusional.

Whether parents are able to be explicit about their differences will become an important factor in determining whether these differences will result in functional or dysfunctional behavior by their child. A schizophrenic family behaves as if there are no differences. Clinically, their interaction appears to operate by means of prohibition and inhibition. Dysfunctioning families typically are those in which the parents lack self-esteem, but in a schizophrenic family the low self-esteem prohibits disagreement, since to disagree is coded as, "You are not good." In such a family, the semblance of agreement protects each person from feeling inadequate, and the sameness fosters the needed illusion of goodness and wholeness.

I am sure that many families operate in this way without anyone developing schizophrenic symptoms, but I expect this would only be possible were there are no outside stresses. I define stress as any required change which is difficult to integrate. And all families know that even a happy event—a new baby, for instance—brings about necessary but temporary stressful changes. Nevertheless, the feeling about the change is tempered by the pleasure in the event. In schizophrenic families, however, any new demand is interpreted as a loss. If the demand is caused by an unhappy event—a catastrophe, a death in the family, a move downward on the social scale, a financial setback—the sense of being unable to cope with a disaster is overwhelming. If a family with a schizophrenic tendency has the luck not to experience a cluster of stresses, however, it is possible that no one will develop untoward symptoms.

All dysfunctioning families have difficulties in handling disagreements, in receiving and giving criticism, and in manifesting individuality, with the result that they will have trouble in expressing themselves as males and females, in handling dependence and independence, and in dealing with authority. The schizophrenic patient reflects the presence of all of these confusions. He acts as though he were both little and big, weak and strong, male and female.

Every person in a family, has a *communication system*, a *premise system*, a *coding system*, and *expectations of outcomes*. *Communication* is the process by which two people give and receiving meaning, and check out that meaning in relation to each other, while *coding* is the meaning a person ascribes to that which he labels. The *premise system* represents the conclusions a person makes about his image of others and the image that he believes others have of him. The system works like a series of mirrors, with the person posing complicated questions: "How do I see me?" "How do I see you?" "How do I see you seeing me?" "How do I see you seeing me seeing you?"

It is impossible for a husband and wife to have identical *premise systems*. They must learn to discover and make room for each other's systems, as well as learn how to handle their differentnesses, so that they will be able to achieve jointly desired outcomes. Explicitness with each other about differentnesses will create an opportunity for the two people to grow and become close to each other. If they cannot accept their differentnesses and cannot be explicit, their unexplored conflicts and confusions will result in a distortion of growth for them and their children. Accepting each other's differences also implies that these two people will make choices on the basis of what is fitting rather than on who is right. If two people react to differentnesses by blaming each other, their conflict will make each one feel isolated, devalued, and incapable.

Perfect communication is obviously impossible. If a person's words and expression are disparate, if he says one thing but seems to mean another by his voice or his gestures, he is presenting what I call an *incongruent manifestation,* and the person to whom he is talking receives a *double-level message.* The whole unsatisfactory interaction is a *discrepancy,* which can be easily solved if people are able to be explicit. "Did you really mean that?" or, "What did you really mean?" or, "You don't look as if you really mean that" are common statements about discrepancies. Usually, the person asked the question is able to be explicit, and the double-level message is clarified.

In a dysfunctioning family, however, the discrepancies are not explicated. The parents manifest themselves incongruently, and their children receive double-level messages. One such manifestation occurs when what is said with words does not fit the way one looks, or the way one sounds. If a woman hurts her child with an unfriendly embrace while saying, "I love you," the child receives a double-level message. Communication analysis deals with this type of discrepancy.

A second type of incongruent manifestation occurs when one looks and sounds in a way that does not fit the situation. Suppose that a parent gives a child a swimming suit and says, "Don't go near the water." Here we have an example of this type of discrepancy, which is relevant to an individual's coding system. A swimming suit is to swim in, but one is told he cannot go to the water. In schizophrenia, the coding system has been badly distorted. If a mother gives her schizophrenic child a swimming suit, he may show this distortion by denying that there is any water in which to swim, or by sitting down on a picture of a lake.

Another incongruent manifestation occurs when how one looks and sounds, and what one does, do not fit with the label that one wears. I call this *role-function discrepancy,* since the function and the label do not match. If a parent asks a three-year-old child to make a decision for the parent, the child has been asked to perform like an adult while he is labeled "child". This puts him in an impossible situation because his perception of what is expected of him gives him an unreal idea of who he is.

All of these discrepancies are present in schizophrenia. They will be found in other types of symptomotology, but in various forms and degrees. Whenever discrepancies exist for a child, he will be unable to grow in a way that will permit him to manifest his independence, his authority or his sexuality.

Discrepancies exist in all human transactions. What distinguishes the functional family from the dysfunctional is the way in which the discrepancies are commented upon. The functioning family is one in which decisions are made in terms of what fits rather than in terms of who is right. The techniques for handling differentnesses are clearly communicated. Decisions are made in terms of time and situation, and each person's view of reality. To illustrate with a trivial example, a child may declare himself in favor of lamb chops for breakfast, but in such a family he will be able to accept the fact that everyone else prefers lamb chops for dinner. Perhaps one parent does not care particularly for lamb chops at any meal, but he or she will be willing at some point to eat them so that the child may enjoy his favorite delicacy. Each person in a functioning family will be able to make choices and decisions for himself in accordance with his age—in terms of his needs, wishes, assets and liabilities—operating within the particular context in which he finds himself. He will be able to take responsibility for his choices and decisions as well as for the resulting outcomes. In other words, each person in a functioning family learns to take charge of himself.

Family therapy is one of the two forms of therapy involving interactional concepts that is in use today. The other one is known as *group therapy*. Since both therapies are oriented around groups, the therapist is able to watch an interaction going on before him among his patients. Group therapy is characteristically made up of patients who are peers. In family therapy there is a group of individuals made up of both peers and nonpeers, the powerful and the powerless, the young and the old. By observing the interaction between the adults and children, and between children and adults, the therapist is able to see where each person is in terms of his present conclusions about himself, and he can also discover more easily the data on which these conclusions are based. Within the family therapy framework, there is, additionally, an opportunity to analyze carefully the internal thoughts and feeling of the family members as they are revealed by questions about how each manifests incongruencies and, further, by analysis of the discrepancies. Treatment consists of the therapist making explicit the presence of a discrepancy, and in learning through explorative questions how each member interprets it and thinks that it came to be, both in other people and in himself.

When he works with an individual, the therapist is part of the interaction, since there are only two people. The therapist cannot easily focus on the interaction between the patient and himself. He hears the patient's report of his internal thoughts and feelings, and his interpretation of those processes, but he must also be able to understand, or to try to understand, what reactions in the patient are a response to the therapist's behavior.

Since it is difficult for any person to make a reliable report on how he himself looks and sounds (simply because no one is able to look objectively at himself), one can only be an authoritative reporter on what he meant or what he felt. A simple illustration is the experience of hearing a tape recording made by oneself. One hears an unfamiliar voice, one's own voice, but others who listen to the tape can easily identify the voice.

The clinician working with one individual has experience in taking clues about how the patient is feeling and thinking from the way he looks and sounds, and in matching that with what the patient says. When the therapist recognizes a discrepancy, he understandably asks himself, "What does the patient really mean?"

The members of the patient's family are in a similar dilemma; that is, they are receiving double-level messages. The therapist's advantage is that he is not bound by the same rules regarding what he may report. He is able to be explicit about what he sees and hears, feels and thinks, and is able, because of this, to comment directly about discrepancies.

For example, a schizophrenic patient in a family therapy session might remark that he had only one eye. The therapist could interpret this statement as the patient's attempt to say that he was only partially understood, that one parent did not understand the other parent, so that they gave him only a partial picture, or that he was unacceptable to his parents because he was incomplete and helpless.

In all dysfunctional families, it is as though there are rules against commenting, and/or commenting directly, and the therapist must try to discover the explicit meaning of a discrepancy; that is, to discover the relationship between what is meant and what is manifest; to discover also the relationship between what is manifest and what was expected, and how what was expected was related to what was happening among all the members of the family.

The clinician working with one patient can observe discrepancies, but he has more difficulty seeing them in himself. It is even possible that he may, without knowing it, manifest incongruently, so that the patient receives double-level messages, thus putting the patient in the same dilemma he faces within his own family. This suggests two advantages in the use of the group. The therapist, by dealing with more than one person at a time, can get a clear picture of how the patient both manifests incongruently and how he reacts to double-level messages. Secondly, if the therapist finds that he is vulnerable to the same kind of discrepancies, he will be able to check himself.

Any idea on the therapist's part that he may be God, mother, or judge makes him apt to send out double-level messages. If he acts as a judge, he will presume to know what is right. If he behaves like a mother, or parent, he will present himself as a nurturer and omnipotent. If he thinks he is God, he will send out messages that he is omniscient. Since no human being is omnipotent or omniscient, and since there is practically nothing about which there is a universal right or a universal wrong, any messages about being God, mother, or judge are double-level in and of themselves. The knotty questions for every therapist is how to be an expert without being omnipotent, omniscient or nurturing, and without recommending what is right or wrong. I think the therapist can avoid this best by using himself as a model for the processes of getting and receiving meaning, while adding his special knowledge about human growth and development, about interaction and about communication.

One of the therapist's chief values is that he was never involved in the initial survival or with the initial blueprints of his patients and he cannot now be. He is a figure from the outside who must be reacted to, since he cannot **not** react to whomever is with him. Every individual has his own processes for integrating an outsider, and observing them helps the therapist to see where each person is in terms of his present level of growth in respect to autonomy, authority and sexuality.

No doubt it is apparent by now that the techniques for family therapy with schizophrenia do not differ from the therapeutic techniques used for other forms of symptomatology. Of course, some symptoms require a greater emphasis on a particular aspect of family integration. In schizophrenia, for instance, the therapist must make a thorough exploration of the patient's premise system so that the patient can be "unhooked" from his present conclusions about himself, which he gained from his respective models, who denied their differentnesses and who presented a picture of perfection and a negation of individuality. More digging is necessary with such a family before they are able to acknowledge the presence of differentnesses and make them explicit.

One of the chief problems in handling schizophrenia, or any symptoms of character disorder, is that the symptom has often been reinforced for years by institutionalization. We are now beginning to take a new look at the diagnosis and treatment of psychological problems, a new look at what we have been doing and how we have been doing it. The implications of the family therapeutic approach for mental health in our society are relevant to prevention, clinical practice, organization of mental health services, the training of clinicians, the understanding of human behavior, and consequently, to symptomatology.

These mental health services are psychiatry, psychology, social work, the counseling services—in short, all the services that employ the people who wear the sign, "I help." Were the family therapeutic approach to be more widely employed, one of the obvious changes would be to arrange the mental health services in a way that would not segment the family. If our agencies could be combined into generic centers for human problems in which the total family unit could be treated, the various specialists could each provide special knowledge, in much the same way that they do in a general hospital. Unfortunately, our present organization of social services helps to create the very problems we would like to alleviate. It is not unusual for one child to be in an institution, another to be seen by a child guidance clinic, and the rest of the family to be on public welfare. In such a predicament there are, in effect, three separate situations each of which has a homeostasis of its own with the result that the family may be further segmented by the treatment. It is also not infrequent for several members of a family to see different therapists, which creates family therapy at the level of the therapists. They get very smart, but what about the patients?

Preventive therapy is of great importance, and the advantage of the family therapeutic approach is that it enables the therapist to identify incipient symptoms in other members of the family. It is possible in the family therapeutic setting to deter the development of pathological processes in other family members. Diagnostic and clinical treatment procedures could be made much more effective if all the family were seen from the beginning. Much time could be saved because there would be no separate, and perhaps conflicting diagnoses, and because duplication of efforts would be eliminated. Diffusion among agencies, as well as segmentation of families, makes it possible to perpetuate a family's dysfunctioning.

If clinicians were trained with the family therapeutic approach as one of their techniques, they would be taught, in addition to psychology, about group interaction, communication processes, and semantics.

The family therapeutic approach suggests that there will be new opportunities to learn about human behavior as it functions both in the internal manifestations of individuals and in their interactions with others. It is to be hoped that these opportunities will make it possible for us to understand more about the complex relationship between human behavior and the development of symptomatology.

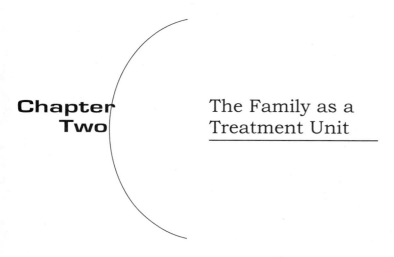

Chapter Two

The Family as a Treatment Unit

Introduction by Stuart Piddocke

When this paper was written, and for what occasion, I do not know. The latest references in the bibliography are dated 1964. This paper stands on its own merits at any time, however, as a crisp and clear statement of a rationale for conjoint family therapy, namely therapy directed not only to individuals but to the family groups of which those individuals are parts. While Satir focuses on the primary triad from which we are all conceived (biological father, biological mother and child), in later writings she extended her ideas to other and more complicated family structures (see chapters 3 and 4, this volume).

This paper invites us to consider each family not as a static structure but as a dynamic process. The family has rules to maintain its way of doing things, but the rules are also tools used by family members to maintain or to change their own positions within the family and to maintain their own identities and survivals, as well as to maintain the family as an ongoing (but not necessarily happy) process. This viewpoint fits neatly with a social-anthropological view of families as part of the ongoing process whereby societies both maintain and change themselves in the midst of that very maintenance. At the same time, this view bears directly on the crucial question concerning the relationships between individual and group behaviors, or micro-systems and macro-systems, which were influencing social-anthropological and sociological thought in the 1960s.

Satir here prescribes a view of therapy as a normative process, namely a process for changing individuals and groups from an unwanted state of being, labeled "dysfunctional" and "deviant", to a desired or better state of being, labeled "functional" and congruent". The functional family fosters the growth of its members in their individual uniquenesses. This is quite different from "adjustment" or "adaptation" in the sense of conformity to group mores. For Satir, genuine therapy necessarily fosters growth.

■ ■ ■

Using the family as a treatment unit in therapy seems to be the inevitable outcome of experience and research in which new knowledge about human behavior has suggested different approaches to the meaning and causation of behavior, and consequently made different treatment procedures possible.

Treating the family as a unit means having all family members present at the same time, in the same place with a single therapist or with male and female cotherapists. The whole family is then viewed and treated as a system originally developed by the male and female adults who are the *architects* of the family.

The symptom of any family member at a given time is seen as a comment on a dysfunctional family system. The wearer of the symptom, the identified patient, is seen as signaling distortion, denial, or frustration of growth. Simultaneously, he is signaling the presence of pain, discomfort or trouble in his relationships with *survival figures.* (Survival figures are those people who have provided and continue to provide nurture, economic support and directing functions for him.)   The major treatment taken in a family therapy is the application of concepts and procedures relating to interaction and communication.

To begin to look at a family system, one can remind oneself that each member of any family is unavoidably committed to the system of his family, if only because that is where he had his beginnings. If the system is an open one, he can use it for his growth. He continues to move in and eventually out of his family system as his maturity develops. Then he himself becomes an architect in developing a further branch of the system, interacting with other people in other situations.

To exist as an open system, the family needs rules that allow it to meet changes openly, directly, clearly and appropriately. The ability for expansion and reshaping is needed for three kinds of changes that inevitably occur because of the nature of life and living. These are:

1. Changes within the individual members: for example, changes that occur between birth and maturity in the use and perception of authority, independence, sexuality and productivity.
2. Changes between family members: for example, between adults and a child from birth to maturity, between husband and wife before they have a child and after the coming of a child, the illness or injury of one, or the advancing age of both husband and wife.
3. Changes that are demanded by social environment: for example, war, a new job, school, neighborhood or country, or new laws.

If the family system is a closed one, the family will handle these inevitable changes by attempting to maintain the status quo, and thus by denying or distorting the change. This creates a discrepancy between the presence of change and the acknowledgement of change, and presents a dilemma that must be dealt with before life and relationships can continue.

Because change must be coped with, a family system that does not have functional ways to assimilate it will have dysfunctional ways. Generally speaking, a system that has rules requiring that the present be seen in terms of the past will be dysfunctional. If the rules of the system can be changed to meet the present, it will become functional. The dysfunctional family, when confronted with change, produces symptoms.

Initially the treatment of behavior problems (of deviant behavior) centered around the person wearing the symptoms. This was true until the advent of child guidance clinics, where the mother was seen along with the child who wore the symptom. Fathers were not discovered until relatively recently in the child guidance clinics. Sometime later, marital counseling or marital therapy (including both husband and wife) was initiated.

Now we have ideas about family therapy that include people as individuals, and in their respective roles: marital, parental, filial, and sibling. Furthermore, we see that the conclusions drawn from experience in the family of origin are connected with the selection of spouse, and with the blueprint for childrearing practices. The symptom is regarded as a report about the individual wearing it, about his family, and about the rules of the family system; and to understand the symptom, one must understand not only the symptom-wearer, but also his family, and the family system.

This means that a symptom such as psychosis in either parent indicates dysfunction in the marital relationship, as well as in child rearing practices. By the same token, symptoms in a child indicate dysfunction in the marital relationship. Thus by seeing the whole family together, we can serve both treatment and preventive functions.

We believe that by observing and learning to understand communication in a family we can discover the rules that govern each individual's behavior. The family system has rules about:

1. Self and manifestation of self, "How I may report."
2. Self and expectation of other, "What I may expect from you."
3. Self and the use of the world outside of the family, "How I may go outside the family."

Family members are not necessarily aware of these rules. We believe the rules are shaped by interactional experience and acquired as each person attempts to survive, grow, get close to others and produce.

Because each person comes into the world without a blueprint for interacting in these ways, he must develop it as he grows from birth. The beginning of this blueprint will, of necessity, be shaped by those who surround him. These are the adults who attempt to insure his survival, through nurture and economic support, through directing his actions, and through providing a model for what he can become.

Most adults have little notion about their importance as models for a child. They behave as though the child sees and hears only that which he is directed to see and hear. If the way in which adults behave with each other and with the outside world, and the way in which the child is asked to behave are incongruent, the child will perceive this. Because the child is confined by the rules about what he may report, by his inability to judge and by his lack of a complete set of reporting symbols, the adult is deluded into believing that he is successfully labeling what the child sees and hears. The parent believes, in other words, that the child does not see or hear that which the parent does not directly direct him to see and hear. In family therapy, however we believe the children's symptoms are a distorted but obvious comment on the discrepancies that they have experienced and are experiencing. The child cannot grow if he must deal with important discrepancies upon which he may not comment openly. Clues to the nature of the discrepancies may be found in the way the family communicates. We approach the analysis of communication by observing and understanding the *means* of communication—the giving, receiving, and checking out of meaning with another, as it is revealed through the use of words, the tone and pace of voice, facial expressions, and body tonus and position. Then we look at the outcome: what actually happens in the communication process, and what kinds of joint decisions or understandings occur.

Next, we examine certain processes to shed light on how these outcomes evolved. We ask:

1. How is the uniqueness and individuality of each person manifested?
2. How are decisions made?
3. How are differences reacted to? In other words, we are attempting to discern the rules for:
   a. Manifesting self and validating to the other uniqueness and individuality.
   b. Making decisions.
   c. Acknowledging the presence of, reacting to, and using differentness.

Our goals in therapy are also related to this analysis of family communication. We attempt to make three changes in the family system. First, each member of the family should be able to report congruently, completely, and obviously on what he sees and hears, feels and thinks about himself and others, in the presence of others. Second, each person should be addressed and related to in terms of his uniqueness, so that decisions are made in terms of exploration and negotiation rather than in terms of power. Third, differentness must be openly acknowledged, and used for growth.

When these changes are achieved, communication within the family will lead to *appropriate outcomes*. Appropriate outcomes are decisions and behaviors that fit the age, ability, and role of the individuals, that fit the role contracts and the context involved, and that further the common goals of the family.

I would like to give you a simple example of the relationship between communication rules and behavior. Suppose that, right now, you are committed to reporting back to me what I have to say, but you can't get my meaning. And there are rules stating that you can't ask about my meaning, for fear of exposing you or me (making a conclusion of badness, sickness, stupidity, or craziness about you or me). If these conditions are present, you will probably lay blame somewhere. There will be three places to point your finger: to yourself, to me, or to the situation.

You will undergo some form of personal discomfort; you will feel anxiety, hostility toward me, and helplessness toward the situation. You may feel anxiety: "I am no good"; hostility: "You are no good"; helplessness: "I am little and weak." And you will probably experience all three feelings roughly in that order—anxiety, hostility, and helplessness. They will have been occasioned by the fact that you could not keep your commitment to yourself. And your inability to keep your commitment to yourself will have been caused by our rules about what kind of questions you can ask.

However if you have rules that permit you to risk exposure and seek clarity in the presence of confusion or lack of clarity, you can save yourself these feelings of anxiety, hostility, and helplessness. Risk requires a perception of your ability to survive in the face of the pain, anger, and hurt in another and the perception that the other will not die from his experience of being pained, angered or hurt. In this context, pain means "I am injured", anger means "You injured me" and hurt means "I don't count".

A direct question is often regarded as a *risk runner*. The infrequent use of direct questions is one of the signals of an inability to communicate in a troubled family; another is the infrequent use of first names.

It should be clear, by now, that I believe that human beings are continually searching to make things fit. Lack of success in making things fit becomes manifest in symptoms. The inability to explore by asking direct questions and making accurate reports does not stop the search; it only makes the search come out in a confused, indirect or unclear way, which may show up in symptoms or inappropriate outcomes.

Thus the analysis of a symptom starts with an analysis of communication, and a documentary of the outcome. Then comes the exploration of the family system, which makes explicit the rules for maintaining the system, and points out the individual processes that implement these rules.

Family therapy centers around the application of concepts of interaction and deals with the present rules and processes of individuals by exploring the family system. Theories relating behavior to interactional process are far from new. Freud used this idea in his treatment of little Hans. Sullivan, Moreno, Ackerman, Lidz, Fleck, Bowen, Bateson, Jackson and Berne, to mention a few, have used interactional concepts to understand human behavior. At present, theories of human behavior that include interactional phenomena are more widely embraced and are getting better understood. Using the family as a treatment unit is a further way to both use and develop the theory.

References

Ackerman, N., Beatman, F., and Sherman, S.W. (1961). Eds. *Exploring the base for family therapy.* New York: Family Service Association.

Brodey, W.M., Bowen, N.M., Dysinger, G. and Basamania, B. (1959). *Some family operations of schizophrenia: A study of five hospitalized families each.* A.M.A. Archives of General Psychiatry, pp. 379-402.

Jackson, D., (1960). *Etiology of schizophrenia.* New York: Basic Books.

MacGregor, R., Ritchie, A.M., Serrano, A.C. and Schuster, F.P. Jr. (1964). *Multiple therapy with families.* New York: McGraw Hill.

Overton, A., Tinker, K.H. (1959). *Casework notebook.* St. Paul, Minn: Family Centered Project.

Satir, V. (1964). *Conjoint family therapy.* Palo Alto, CA: Science and Behavior Books.

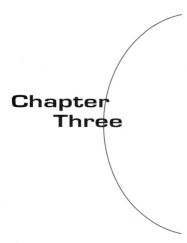

Chapter Three

Family Systems and Approaches to Family Therapy

Introduction by Gloria Taylor

Readers then and now cannot help but feel the excitement as Satir refers to the advances and insights into family therapy that were happening in 1966. It was as though Satir could see into the future and predict that the discoveries of those times would become anchors for the future understandings of families and family therapies. As she says, "We are living in a very magnificent time as far as human beings are concerned."

The experimentation of those times, as she points out, was to reveal aspects of the family members' ties to one another, the specificity of these ties and how the parts of the family are larger than the whole. Thus, she sets the stage for interventions that would change interactive patterns to the betterment of the whole. Satir's excitement and passion are evident in the opening and closing paragraphs of this presentation. She closes with " We are at a very exciting time in looking at relationships" and, " It is exciting for me, for others and I hope it is for you, too" This was true in 1966 and is true in 2008. It is as though we are looking back at a very personal glimpse of a visionary. Such a privilege!

Current students of family systems theory will appreciate Satir's view of the changes in diagnosis and treatments over time. Then patients were labeled as psychiatric and treated with drugs, electric shock and insulin regressions in order to manage their "crazy" behavior. Satir saw these treatments as punitive. This no-

tion of punishment becomes central to her growth model versus the prevailing threat—reward model.

Satir had an infectious sense of humor. Many moments in her live presentations and demonstrations of family work were sprinkled with the spontaneous sharing of pictures in her head. She would lift the tension of the moment when required with her lively sense of humor. The high value she placed on humor made the space safe and intimate. As she points out, there was an early premise that a child's behavior was influenced by the mother. "Fathers were discovered later." How could the listener or reader not smile when she says this?

Satir also suggests that "children were there to help a husband and wife get along together". Family systems theory acknowledges the invisible positions and tasks that are unwittingly assumed by children and offers new ways of seeing and intervening in family therapy based on this perspective.

Outstanding in this piece is Satir's careful separation of the label from the person. She had the privilege of being a colleague of Gregory Bateson and Murray Bowen. Along with others, these courageous clinicians veered from the views of the times and offered new and far more useful ways of seeing who we are at deeper intricate levels of the self.

Systems theory was developed in science (Bertalannfy) but for the first time it has applications in the family. As Satir points out, language for family applications was unsatisfactory at the time, so she brilliantly offers a glossary of terms at the end of this paper—so endearing!!

Satir goes on to offer a precise description of communication between receiver and sender and how intricately this affects self-esteem. It seemed to her worthwhile to scrutinize more carefully. One has the sense that she was on to something revolutionary long before the self/other context was a concept. It is a concept in the making.

Further on in the article, "I believe that our whole physical system is made up of so many parts with which we are not in connection …" reflects Satir's awareness and attention to our inner beings, later metaphorically depicted as an iceberg.

People have sophisticated ways of taking care of themselves. They develop coping strategies learned in the family, which are largely informed by tacit rules. Here one can see how the relevance of family rules, particularly rules about commenting, are identified, how family rules are made covert and how expectations *are informed as well. What was learned at a very early stage of life is bound to inform perceptions, expectations and behaviors in adults. As Satir subtly points out, explanations we make to ourselves in stress situations are similar to what has been done over the ages to explain deviations.*

Satir believed that human beings are not innately destructive and that family therapy with a systems' view could and would prevent relational disasters. At this point in time there has been much research that confirms her hope and excitement. How fortunate we are to be able to drift back over time with this great visionary teacher.

■ ■ ■

I would like to put together some things and some ideas that have proved very interesting and exciting to me, and, I think, to others in this country and elsewhere. I am connected with working people and their problems by working through the medium of the family unit. Because I believe we are living in a very magnificent time as far as human beings are concerned, I would like to trace for you what I think are the origins of both their growth and change. Many new things are coming up—social psychiatry, community psychiatry, the influences of existentialism and of self-actualization. There is a spirit of experimentation around, which is always exciting. Let me develop some of the ideas that I think lead to the understanding of the family unit, which I see as a step in evolvement more than any particular form of therapy, as opposed, for instance, to working with an individual or a group.

I want to cover hundreds of years of history very quickly. The origins of any of the therapeutic entities we deal with at present, it seems to me, come from *the witch, the pauper, the idiot, the sick person,* and *the criminal.* Our present areas of interest have evolved from these five kinds of people. We got psychiatry from *the witch,* criminology from *the criminal,* medicine from *the sick person,* social work from *the pauper,* and psychology from *the idiot.* It is not exactly one to one, but all of these entities were, at one point, perceived as deviations, where causality was unknown. From these, however, came the first diagnostic categories. And then, as in all diagnostic categories, a series of causations were suggested, as well as a series of therapies. Starting from the labeling and the causation of deviations and their treatment, we look back and see that the first theories of causation about deviation were unknown, but the treatment was death by indirection or by direction.

I am going back many years to try to develop these three lines: the *labeling*, the *causation*, and the *treatment* within this framework of deviation. I want to make some sense out of where we are today. People were not content to look upon deviation and the fact that its causes were unknown. Human beings are a curious lot, and they try to figure things out. As they began to look at these deviations, one of their first ideas about causation was some kind of unknown infiltration from without, some kind of magic at that particular point. We have in some cultures today, certain religious beliefs that would be used for this. As the years progressed, it was thought that perhaps it was not all magic; maybe it had something to do with what you were like when you were born—your genetic heritage. If it was something that you were born with, there was not much you could do about it; you had to be content to endure it. However, society might try to segregate the genetically unwhole people and place them somewhere else.

We had by this time, then, three theories about causation: unknown, infiltration from outside, and genetic. Treatment could be death, or it could be separation of some sort.

As the years went on, it looked as if a person's behavior had something to do with his will; that is, he was an "ornery cuss," and that was his trouble. As the idea developed that man was just an "ornery cuss," it seemed that if this were the cause of his behavior, one way of taking care of it was to punish him. Now we had another form of treatment. It looks like man explored a little bit more and got the idea that perhaps where a person lived had something to do with how he behaved. The natural and logical conclusion to that was to move him to a place with different surroundings; thus custodial care came into being, and we have many residuals of that.

Later, it looked as though behavior had something to do with some part of a person that motivated him, but was out of sight of his awareness. This was, of course, the unconscious. The treatment for that was to discover the unconscious and try to help a person by putting him more in charge of himself. Psychoanalysis was one of the main tools for that particular form of treatment. Then it seemed as though the way one person behaved had something to do with the person with whom he was interacting, and the theory of interpersonal behavior was born. Therefore, it seemed sensible to treat the interpersonal relationship and the milieu.

In a brief way I have covered the general kinds of theories of causation and treatment—and these were all one-to-one things. Different ideas came into being such as interpersonal theory, which Sullivan wrote about in the 1920's and we saw the rise of something called group therapy in with Moreno, Slavson and some of the others. With this came the idea treating an individual with his peers who were in the same spot. This group treatment, or treatment within a peer group, was based upon one principle: Changes in the behavior of an individual were brought about through interpersonal operation. Before World War II, these two ways of treating were invoked: the individual and the group.

At the beginning of the century, there also developed something called child guidance clinics, which provided the first form of treatment based on an interpersonal relationship. These used the unit of the mother and the child on the premise that the child's behavior was influenced by what the mother did. Fathers were discovered later. We had two uses of the interpersonal relationship, that is, that which was perceived in child guidance, and that which was worked out in group therapy.

After World War II came another kind of treatment, known as marital counseling, for the husband and wife pair. For the most part, marital counseling was not brought into the profession by psychiatrists, social workers, and such, but rather by clergymen, sociologists, and other people outside of the usual (forgive the expression) *mental ill health* disciplines. I use that term because all of us in the psychiatry, social work, or psychology professions are mental-ill-health specialists. We had another form of the mental treatment unit then, the husband and wife.

So, at this point we have the picture of how to treat an individual, how to treat groups of individuals, the mother-child unit, and the husband-wife unit. If you look at this in terms of a family, you will see that there are only two other units present in the family, but still left out: the father-child unit and the sibling unit. So if we add the sibling unit and the father-child unit to the mother-child unit and the husband-and-wife unit, we have all the units in a family.

We had the beginnings, if we put them all together, of what would go into a family. To take a little further look, along came the idea that children were there to help, in an indirect way, a husband and wife to get along together. Also, running through all of this was an idea that people could be taught how to take on marital and parental responsibilities. So much, then, for the evolvement up to the time of World War II.

There was also a psychiatric entity called schizophrenia, which had been around for a long time and which happened to be a label that, in years past usually meant that nothing much could be done for people to whom it was applied. Occasionally, there were scattered reports of improvement or recovery but, by and large, in the treatment of that entity called schizophrenia, the prognosis was not very good. After the last war, some curious people began to think about how a person who was labeled a schizophrenic might look to his own family. Gregory Bateson, an anthropologist who was associated with us at the Mental Research Institute, was one of the people who became curious as to what the whole family looked like if it contained someone with this label. He began his studies in 1954, and around the same time, Murray Bowen, who was at the National Institute of Mental Health, hospitalized whole families just to look at this situation. Some interesting things emerged in the studies of the schizophrenic and his family—when I say "schizophrenic," I mean somebody who has that label. There seemed to be a repetitious and predictable pattern, a direct link, between what the labeled person was presenting and the family of which he was a part. This excited people because, again, theories of behavior ranged all the way from the unknown and genetics to the other things I have mentioned. The idea developed that maybe we had something new that would shed some light on the behavior of a person—in this instance, the behavior of a schizophrenic. It was not a very long step then to looking at all other kinds of behavior to see if the behavior of any individual could be linked to the system of which he was a part.

In the early days we did not talk much about systems. We just knew that we were seeing a series of patterns that certainly seemed to have a type of link. Also, it appeared, that every group of essential ingredients that must belong together in order to emerge with a single outcome formed a system. The parts had to work together in some kind of organized, orderly, sequential form, which began to develop a rhythm and a balance in order to obtain the outcome that the particular ingredients are designed to do. It began to look as though each family developed a system from its ingredients, a system that somehow kept the whole family in balance.

This was a crude beginning, that is, the observation that families were systems which worked like cars. In biology we were well acquainted with systems; it seemed that a similar thing went on in families. At the Mental Research Institute we had done a great deal of work trying to find out about family systems, trying to see how they worked, and trying to see what kinds of intervention one needs to change a system that is not functioning toward growth to one that was. This brought a new idea into focus, because when we tried to determine whether or not the behavior of an individual was healthy, we used one set of criteria. But when we looked at behavior in relation to a system, these criteria did not fit and we had to look at something else. The words that would describe a functioning person would not necessarily describe a functional system. We had no words to talk about human systems, and we had to devise a new language. I am not satisfied with the language we have worked out for talking about systems, but I think we will learn more about it.

The Mental Research Institute was founded in 1959 to study the relationship of individual behavior to the system of which it was a part. When we started to explore this, we had to review certain things that we knew about the development of a person. And then the *system* idea became even more sensible. All of you probably know, when you think about it, that you arrived where you are right now and became the person you are at this moment because of a three-person learning system: a male and a female forebear and yourself. If you did not actually have one of these persons on the premises, their images were on the premises. So we knew that every individual becomes the product of a three-person learning system: a male adult and a female adult, who are his parents, and himself. We also knew, when we reminded ourselves, that every child comes into this world with only ingredients to grow and not a blueprint already developed. There are no cases on record where there was a little bag of directions about how to grow and develop. The important thing we all recognized was that this blueprint had to be drawn as the child went along. Obviously, the blueprint depended upon the way in which the male and the female adult handed down to their child, the directions for how he was to grow.

On the face of it, that sounds easy. A couple of adults put their heads together and work out, or write out, a blueprint for the kids. However, it does not seem to work that easily in practice. When two adults get together, even though they are the parents of a child, they are not always in agreement about what makes for the best kind of blueprinting. They are not always able to communicate their messages to the child, or to each other, so there is no particular guarantee that a child will get a clear message from his parents about how he should grow and develop. However, as we looked at how adults pass on to the child their ideas for the child's development, we came onto this very important thing: communication.

Communication has been known about for a long time; in mass communication everybody is connected, that is, knows something about it. But we defined this a little bit further. We said that communication was a two-way street and that it took place between a sender and a receiver, and that whether or not the communication came across depended both upon the sender and upon the receiver. Every child has two senders, the male adult and the female adult. I don't know whether this is lucky or unlucky, but he may also have some other senders around, like grandparents, or aunts. There are at least two senders, but the child is only one receiver.

We therefore concocted this idea: Suppose that you were a radio receiver and you were being sent signals from two different stations—neither of which knew that the other one was sending and they had to come in on the same wave length. You know what happens with that? You get static. You also had a commitment on the receiving end regardless of what was going on or what the reality was, to make sense of the signals and to use them as though they fit. This was especially true if there was a rule that the sender and receiver could not comment to one another, or that the receiver could not send anything back, or that he could not even comment on the fact that what he was sent does not fit. In a rather homely analysis, it looked to us as if every child was involved in such a situation and dependent upon it for the development of his self-concept. All of us who had any knowledge from working with individuals knew that the picture a person had of himself, and the feeling of self-worth that he had, was going to be very important in determining how that person would behave, how he would grow, how he would feel, and how he would act. It seemed then that it would be worthwhile to scrutinize more carefully the operation between the male adult and the female adult in the interests of their child.

One of the things that we discovered, contrary to what had

been thought originally, was that not everything the child got from the parent was what the parent intended to give. (We went through a period when it was quite clear that all the bad things of the world were related to mothers—the bad mothers that did all the harm—and we had techniques that dealt with that.) But we found that there was not much relationship between what the parent intended and what the child received. Neither was there much relationship between what one parent sent out and what the other sent out, particularly if the two were not aware that they could send out different messages. We learned that the knowledge of the child, in contrast to the intentions of the parent toward this child, would not necessarily be refused by the child. For the first time, someone could look at assistance outside *blame frame.*

There is a difference between seeing how things work and finding blame or credit for the way things work. And I would say at this point in time that all over the world and in all groups that I work with, when people are trying to explain causes, they still get into the blame frame. It is very difficult not to do this without raising defenses, without making people feel badly, without making people fight, and fight in a purposeless kind of way.

If it were true that the messages of the adults were not necessarily communicated to the child and received by him as intended, then we needed to look at this more carefully. In doing so, we came upon some very simple things. (I am quite convinced that it is the simple things in the world that we overlook most often, and, if I am an expert in anything, I would consider myself an expert in the obvious that most likely gets overlooked.) We discovered that it is quite possible for us, in sending messages, to give the receiver clues that we are not aware of giving. There is a very simple explanation: When we are preoccupied with our inner selves we do not recognize what we are presenting outside. But the children do. We discovered that parents had the delusion that their children only heard what their parents intended them to hear and only saw what they intended them to see. We discovered also that parents gave out what are known as *double-level messages.*

This was one of the contributions that Gregory Bateson made, and I want to tell you about a *double-level*, because we're *double-leveling* all the time. Double-leveling in itself is not pathological. These messages gave us clues that the parents' intent was not received by the child. Let me give you the definition of a double-level message. Suppose that I announce, with a big grin on my face, that the building is burning down. There is something here that does not quite fit. Now, if you are in my presence when I have a big grin on my face and I say to you, "The place is burning down," you are in a dilemma. If you take your message from my smile, there is something funny about this. Yet, you are not supposed to have joy and pleasure when the place is burning down. If you listen to my words about the place burning down, then what are you going to do with my smile? This is a double-level. Or, suppose I get a bad pain while I am with a friend. I do not want my friend to know that I am in pain because we have other things to do, but she observes that my facial muscles get stiff and taut, and says, "How are you feeling?" If I reply, "Fine," I am really saying, "You don't have to look at my pain, we can go on with what we are doing." But, seeing my face, my friend may very well conclude that I am an idiot, that I am lying to her, that I do not consider her enough of a friend that I can level with her, or other things of this sort. These are double-levels again.

Double-levels come about without people knowing it, and in my opinion, there is nothing pathological about that. It is pathological when double-levels are not commented upon or acknowledged in some way by those to whom they are directed. Explanations can give a chance, at least, for an understanding of what does not fit. Many times in talking to groups, people want to make the point that it is bad if you give out double-levels. I do not think you can live without them. I believe that our whole physical system is made up of so many parts with which we are not in connection that we are unaware of a great many of our clues.

As speakers, each of us relates more to what is inside than what is outside; as listeners, we are more aware of what is presented to our outsides and take our clues from what we see and hear. If we cannot comment on the clues, we must determine for ourselves the reasons for the discrepancies. Now, if you happen to be a person with low self-esteem, you probably are going to interpret a discrepancy in some impulsive way. You may conclude that it is a lie, or some form of sick, bad, stupid, or crazy behavior. Unless you can check it out, you are likely to retain a false interpretation of the discrepancy.

Children come into the world unequipped to give any kind of specific feedback. They usually do not learn to talk until the age of twelve months or beyond. For those twelve months of a child's life, he had to interpret, on his own, whatever discrepancies he has envisaged or experienced with his parents. By the time the child is talking, he already has a wealth of clues defined; he has a set of expectations to which he will give words later on, much to the surprise of the adults.

We were interested in looking at what we thought would help us with the mystery of how a person with good intentions, who is right and loving, could give out faulty messages to a child. (I am sure that you have noticed that there is not much relationship between love, niceness, and hard work among the people who have problems in your family.) So how could it be that a person, who was well intentioned, loving and bright, still managed to have children who were not growing properly? I think the answer is in not knowing that adults are capable of giving double-levels and that the child has to make some kind of sense out of them. I sometimes wonder how any child, especially if he is around many adults in his first year of life, manages some kind of integration with himself.

One of the things that has been very interesting at the Mental Health Institute is the use of video tapes. I felt that it was most important to acquaint families with the fact that the way they thought they looked and sounded was not the way they really looked and sounded. What somebody else got from them was not necessarily what they thought was there. Another myth was that one should always be one hundred percent in control of the way he manages himself. It was easy to dispel that kind of expectation with television, but you cannot run around with your tape recorder all the time. We looked for other ways in which a person could find out that he did not always look and sound as he thought he did. If you do not believe me, go home tonight, walk in the door and tell the first person you see to look at you, and then you tell him what you think he saw. Describe fully your eyes and your nose, what your ears are doing, and what the muscles in your neck are doing, and whether you are red or not. Then compare the picture with his view. This is a descriptive exercise. Nobody is telling you that anything is wrong with you; you are just comparing pictures.

There is another thing that you can do. Very few of us have ever seen ourselves as we really look. Go to your mirror and put on a name tag. Look in the mirror. You will see that your name tag is backwards. If you have never seen yourself on a video tape or in moving pictures, you have been running around all your life with a delusion of what you look like. You have been comparing feedback with a delusion instead of with reality. Similarly, the first time you hear your voice on a tape recorder, you say to yourself, "That is not me, my voice is lower than that, or, it is higher than that." But everybody else says that it is exactly the way you sound. A very simple physics principle governs that little discrepancy: sound that originates in the same orifice is heard differently than the sound that comes from outside of that orifice. Again, we have the possibility for delusions and I use *delusion* in a nice sense because I am not afraid of them. I used to be, but I am not any more. People run around with some mistaken ideas that they know what they look like, what they intend to say, and what they sound like. There is a fourth part to this belief: whatever they intend to look like and sound like, they mistakenly believe they do look like and sound like.

Much of what we have developed in the way of treatment intervention has been based upon these kinds of things—the ways in which the child receives his messages initially on how to develop his blueprints. There are many ways of doing it, and you can see now how many traps there would be for a child in getting messages from his mother and father within the expectations that I have described. If this is accompanied by the rule against commenting upon what the child sees and hears when he can talk, you can see how the child could continue his early misconceptions of what was intended without his parents being aware of them. Maybe this is so until the child goes to school, when suddenly there comes some demand on his growth which he cannot see, and then the whole story comes out.

I would like to make one other point in looking at the development of the child: We were all children once. It sounds a little facetious when I say it, but many adults forget this—that they were once children, and that their origins were as children. Because we were all children, we all have ideas about how children should be different. All adults have in their minds a picture of the ideal child. And from where do they get that ideal child? Where did you get your ideas of what your ideal child is like? You got them from what you were not, from what your parents did not do properly, and from how they told you you ought to be. Everybody wants things to fit their ideals. So each adult applies these same things to his child when he comes along, and we think this is one of the ways that social heredity takes place. It seems that because of the ways in which rules about commenting are made in the family, people develop rules for themselves—whether or not they can comment, whether they can criticize, or whether they can make loving comments. And the less the ability and freedom to comment, the more likely are going to be the distortions, inhibitions, and prohibitions about what people can comment on later.

People can grow to adulthood with rules that permit them to comment only on certain things, and the rest of it may be just imagined or believed, even though it may not even be in reality. Then people get married. Their marriage relationship may be founded upon their ideals of what should be, which can be filled in easily if you do not ask for reality to be validated. It is very easy for a woman to believe that a man must always be a leader, because her father was not the leader and her mother said that he should be. Her idea then is that the man tells her what to do. But his telling her what to do in the courtship period means that he always had an idea about where the two can go. Later on, the same things happen, except it feels different. What at one point in time felt like a strong man taking care of her, later feels like a bully trying to squash her. Where would she get such delusions? Not only from inside herself, but also from when he once said, "Let's go to the movies," and she said, "No." He said, "Yes," and she felt that he was a strong man. So this is her fantasy, and she begins relating herself to him in terms of this fantasy. As long as you do not comment upon it, you do not have to break up your fantasy: you can continue.

However, at some time reality presents itself, and it is no longer possible to continue life with a fantasy. We think that a symptom breaks out when the reality can no longer sustain the fantasy. We have quite a bit of evidence to get us on this track, and I think this is a very fruitful way of beginning. Human beings, we find, do not give up easily. Even when the woman should decide her husband is trying to squash her, she will still try to make sense of it in some way and keep her symptom, because people do not give up easily. Things begin to develop such as, "I'm unlovable, now here is the evidence." Then she withdraws more, and of course he sees that he is being withdrawn from, so there must be something wrong with him. Then we get back to the magical thinking: he was born that way, lived with the wrong people, got a little man in his head telling him what to do. These begin to be some of the explanations that take place. Isn't it interesting that the explanations these people make at this point in time are so similar to what we did, over the ages to the present, to explain deviations?

We are at a very exciting time in looking at these relationships. First of all, there is evolvement in the ideal self-concept within the family system, and the kinds of communications patterns that go into it. Right now, we are working on some ideas about child rearing by having adults know more. It is much easier to know about communication than it is to know about your self-concept, and apparently it is not so defense producing. We are working on ways to make it possible for young parents to do a different kind of job regarding what they pay attention to in rearing their children. We are working also on the *well family service*, which we think will develop into a preventive device. We see now that every family has a predictable system of operations and a set of expectations and predictions. These expectations and predictions are part of the evolvement of the self-concept of each person involved. It will be expressed through behavior and through communication. If we put all these together, we can begin to know something about helping with behavior that is on the road to some kind of destruction. We hope that many people will help us with this. It is exciting for me, I think that it is for others, and I hope that it is for you, too.

Selected Concepts and Terminology

Conjoint: *Con* treating all the members as contributors to a single system of which each member is also a receiver, instead of treating one in the service of another
Joint having all family members together at one time in one place with the same therapist
Emphasis is on perception, interaction, transaction, and communication instead of intrapsychic phenomena

Homeostasis: A process by which the family balances forces within itself to achieve unity and working order

Self-Concept: Internal perception of self
Self-Esteem: The value a person thinks and feels

A sense of mastery over self and environment based to large extent on how he sees other people seeing him

Congruent: Things fit

Congruent Manifestation: Words, voice tone, facial expression, body movement give a clear, explicit message

Incongruent: Things don't fit

Incongruent Manifestation: Person's words and expression are disparate—says one thing and seems to mean another by his voice and/or gestures
Results in a discrepancy

Dilemma: Situation presenting two or more solutions; neither totally satisfactory idea is to reach compromise between self and other

Integration: Person can see, feel, think and hear; understands what he sees, feels, thinks and hears; is free to report or comment and can handle the feedback

Functional: Integrated—person feels freedom to comment or report and can handle feedback

Dysfunctional: Not integrated—person doesn't feel free to comment or report on incongruencies and cannot handle feedback

Differentness: Covers whole area of individuality; how each person is innately different from every other person

Growth: Is possible when the survival, intimacy, productivity and making sense and order life needs are met; use of things and experience

Therapeutic

Process: Creation of an open system: making person
                      aware of how and why he makes choices;
                      extending of awareness; developing new
                      methods of coping

Coping: Dealing with and balancing the require-
                      ments of you, me and the context at a par-
                      ticular point in time under a given set of
                      circumstances

Hope: Person feels he has opportunity for growth

Trust: Quality that allows a person to assert his
                      thoughts, wishes, feelings and knowledge
                      without being afraid of being destroyed, in-
                      volved or obliterated by the other or convey-
                      ing this to another person

Change Artist: Anyone who wears the label "I help"

Life Needs: Survival, intimacy, productivity, making sense
                      and order

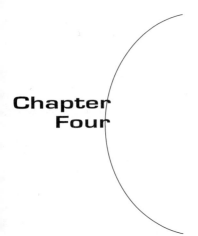

Chapter Four

The Growing Edge of Myself as a Family Therapist

Introduction by Pindy Badyal

In reading this article, I was struck by Satir's eagerness to grow and evolve as a therapist. As a family therapist myself, I am inspired by her emphasis on our own continuing growth as therapists. Her ability to connect with people, her willingness to be creative, her focus on positive resources of individuals, as well as her courage to take risks, make her a true forerunner of family therapy. Her curiosity to learn about the capacity of the human spirit to survive and thrive, combined with her keen interest in accessing people's internal resources and her ability to connect with individuals at a deep level, enabled her to be a truly gifted and skilled family therapist.

Satir begins the article by providing a brief overview of how in 1951 she "inadvertently...stumbled into what later came to be called family therapy." The article vividly portrays her innovative style of working with clients and their families. During the early 1950s, while other practitioners worked from a psychodynamic perspective focused on pathology, Satir used creative therapeutic tools to zero in on the positive resources of the individuals with whom she worked. Consequently, new possibilities and new vistas were opened up for her. She joined forces with Don Jackson and Jules Riskin and founded the Mental Research Institute in Palo Alto. Satir was interested in further developing and refining her theory of self-esteem. In 1964, when Satir went to Esalen, she became better acquainted with other practitioners and their modalities of therapy, *including Fritz Perls and Gestalt Therapy, Eric Berne and Transactional Analysis, and Al Lowen's Bioenergetics. Satir was indeed a true collaborator; she worked collaboratively not only with her clients but her colleagues.*

Satir's conviction to emphasize the importance of self-esteem deepened as she continued her work with families. In addition to seeking to advance her theory of self-esteem, she went on to create various therapeutic tools including the survival coping stances, simulated family, family reconstruction, and family of origin map, all of which are still very popular among family therapists. Her work with families also led her to conclude that the therapeutic alliance was an important factor in promoting change for clients. She notes, "...I see the relatedness to what I do as potentially able to foster evolvement of each self in the family, create nurturing interrelationships in the family..." It is noteworthy that the importance of the therapeutic alliance is attracting the attention of many contemporary scholars, clinical practitioners and researchers.

This article would be helpful for family therapists who are interested in expanding their repertoire of therapeutic tools in working with families. A wide variety of therapeutic strategies are described. Satir's acute awareness of people's verbal and nonverbal interactions is impressive. Her intuitive ability to connect with her clients at a deeper level is exceptional. Her belief that a strong therapeutic alliance is critical in allowing clients to begin the risk of personal change and growth continues to be very relevant in the therapeutic arena. To be a successful family therapist, one must make contact with each family member and continually focus on the verbal and nonverbal interactions among and between the various family members. This is very evident throughout the article.

■ ■ ■

Twenty-five years ago, in January, 1951, I inadvertently saw my first family with intent to "cure." I had literally stumbled into what later came to be called family therapy. At that time I had eight years of experience as a psychoanalytically-oriented psychotherapist working with individuals. It took a long time for the patient to make changes, but on the whole the results were good —so much so that I dared to enter private practice. I had had six years of elementary and secondary teaching experience and eight additional years struggling to help people by working with them individually.

At the time I was working with a 24-year-old woman who had come to me with the diagnosis of "ambulatory schizophrenia." After about six months of bi-weekly sessions and much improvement, I got a call from her mother threatening to sue me for alienation of affection. For whatever reason that day, although I clearly heard her threat, I heard something else: the plea under the threat. And under that threat was hurt. I responded to that and invited her to join her daughter and me—an invitation which she promptly accepted.

Within a matter of minutes after the mother joined the interview, my patient began to behave as she had when I first saw her. All the seeming growth had evaporated before my eyes. I went through many emotions very quickly—disbelief, anger, self-criticism—until finally my computer tipped me off to stop blaming and become an observer of what was happening. After I collected myself, I stopped listening to the words and started watching the nonverbal clues going back and forth between the two, and I began to notice repetitive patterns emerging. It seemed that the daughter had different clues to deal with in her mother than she did with me. It further seemed that the pattern established with her mother was more powerful than with me. Much later, I theorized that, of course, it would be that way because she and her mother had a survival basis for their relationship that was not true for me. Also later, I became aware that, until somehow the patient became an initiator as well as a responder, she would be hopelessly a victim of other people's initiation.

I didn't know it then, but I was at the beginning of an understanding of how human behavior takes place by a response to current interactional clues and how eventually this evolves into a predictable pattern. Nor did I understand how this, in turn, weaves itself into a system, to serve the needs of survival. I was also quite aware that I was violating the psychoanalytical rule: "Don't see relatives." Then, somewhere within a period of five or six weeks of seeing mother and daughter together, it occurred to me that there just might be a father somewhere. I inquired and sure enough there was a father.

Once more I was violating a cardinal rule, because in those days only mothers were seen to be in the pathological picture. Father accepted my invitation to join us. After his entrance, the patterns widened to include more movements, and these movements were compatible with what I had seen with the mother and daughter. I didn't realize it at the outset, but I was looking at the *double-bind phenomenon* that only later was to be named by Gregory Bateson and Don Jackson. This pattern came to be commonly associated with families where there was a schizophrenic member. The picture of this family was completed when my patient's "good" brother came into the interview. I was certainly "traveling by the seat of my pants!"

But things worked out well. I think that what saved me, and gave me the courage to go on, was that I forgot about curing and simply observed and commented on what I saw. The theorizing came later. There was absolutely nothing in the literature then except Freud's case of little Hans and Sullivan's interpersonal theories. No one that I knew was seeing anyone except on an individual basis. I was quite alone. Furthermore, by this time, I was totally dependent on private practice. To live, I had to have "satisfied customers;" to remain respected in my profession, I could have no suicides or homicides; and to respect myself, I certainly could not violate any patient to serve my own ends. The profession at that time was heavily psychoanalytic and I was trying to respect that, too. Besides, that was the only approach I had; the only tools I had were psychoanalytic ones.

I began to invite the families of other patients in to see if there were similar trends. There were. I was in the position of observing things that I neither fully understood, nor did I know how to deal with them creatively.

Out of this experience came a new tool, something I called a *family life fact chronology.* With the whole family present I would take what was essentially the story of the events in the lives of all the family members—who was where, when, and what happened. This was not the social history; it was a chronological history. I learned to take facts, which emphasized developmental events and traumatic episodes. I started out with the simple idea that if I took the calendar time period from the birth of both parents to the present date, and filled it in year by year, I could get some feel for the continuity of the family. It gave me an opportunity to find out how each person experienced the chronological events.

During the course of this phase of inquiry, I learned how very little family members actually knew about their facts, how very diverse were the views of family members and, in many cases, how they differed about the facts. Perhaps the biggest result of the family-life fact chronology was that, although it concerned the past, it did in fact create a currently alive situation where members began to communicate with one another—adding, correcting, informing, confronting. Besides getting helpful information for me to understand the past, and to clue in to some of the forces with which the families wrestled currently, it provided continuity for the family. This chronology became a reliable way to place the family in time and place. I tried to present this to the family with the feeling of adventure. I showed as much interest in what happened positively as I did to the negative happenings. My main thrust was to keep the family members' attention focused on how they responded individually to the information.

In retrospect, I feel that the real pay-off for this tool was when I saw that it turned out to be a believable, understandable means of authentically providing the family with a means of interacting in the present. I began to get real clues about the fantasies and expectations that each had of the other, which without clarification, stood as fact. Unraveling this became the basis of my present communication theory.

After doing perhaps several hundred of these myself, I began to see the emergence and effect of systems in the family, and I was given more confidence as a result. This tool became the basis for what I now use to prepare a person to do his *family reconstruction,* another tool I have developed. I began to understand how the perceptions gained very early in life tended to become the yardstick around which the person measures the world and others, as though his childhood context had not changed. This was not necessarily a new idea. I called these old learnings. What was new about this concept was that I was able to help the person bring himself up to date and to perceive the context he was actually in, without threat, rather than to continue to perceive things as though he were still in an earlier context. I could only develop this after I began to work with families in groups. I did it through a role-playing process. I made the assumption that whatever we carry around with us as a learning from the past is a personal construct—the best we had—but it may bear little or no relation to what actually happened. Even so, we see through the lens of our constructs. They are in us.

I had been taught to view behavior in pathological terms, but as I began to see families, I began to see their responses much more in terms of relevant, current self-esteem needs, which were both in and out of awareness. At that point in time I was giving the psychiatric nomenclature and Freud's theory of the unconscious some very careful scrutiny. In teaching residents at the Illinois State Psychiatric Institute from 1955 to 1958, I really had to look at, and think about, what I was teaching because residents have a way of asking questions I had never thought of. This experience made it necessary for me to really develop my theoretical base, and thus new vistas were opened up for me.

After joining with Don Jackson and Jules Riskin to found the Mental Health Research Institute in Palo Alto, it remained for me to develop the whole concept of *communication*, which today I view as the energy that keeps the human system going. The burning questions became: What kind of system leads to healthy functioning and what kind leads to unhealthy functions? What are the manifest clues that one uses to judge?

Once I more fully understood how a verbal message actually contains two messages, one verbal and the other nonverbal, I was able to see that the two messages could contradict one another. It was a short step to connect this with my developing self-esteem theory; that is, the main thrust of people's relationship was to survive psychologically. Further, there was the emerging idea that behavior was largely out of the person's awareness. What could I do to help the person bring his own behavior into awareness and thus give him the opportunity to decide whether or not he wanted to make changes?

Putting together what I knew of continuity, communication and self-esteem, the *simulated family tool*, the *communication stances* and *games* followed in rapid succession.

Incidentally, most of my tools have developed from something accidental or some need of the moment. For example, my version of the simulated family developed when I was hired to do a demonstration of family therapy for the Colorado Welfare Conference in 1962-1963. Somewhere along the line someone had neglected to get a family with whom I was to work. When I found this out, and when I got over the panic that ensued, I said to myself, "All right, Virginia, if you are so smart about family systems, you ought to be able to make a simulated family." Somewhere from the back of my head came the design. I tried it and it not only worked, it became the model that I have used ever since. I use this when I work with groups of families. I put students who are learning family therapy in different kinds of simulated families; I also use this model when I do family reconstruction. Experiencing being in a simulated family helps one to understand the power of a system in a hurry and at the same time introduces one to the universals in family systems.

When it came to the communication stances, one day I was thinking about all the different kinds of communication responses I had seen, and they categorized themselves in my mind in five different categories, which bore a neat, almost uncanny resemblance to what I had observed in people over the years. These five kinds of behaviors all seemed to be aimed toward survival, and, in addition, seemed to be out of the awareness of the individuals exhibiting them. Now I believe that it is perfectly possible for a person to have a dissonance between his inside feelings and his outside expression. I called that *incongruence*. That was not a new idea either. What I added was a graphic, physical picture.

Since I believe that pictures speak louder and clearer than words, I made body pictures of what I now call the communication stances. I had noticed certain kinds of physical postures and the affect that accompanied certain kinds of verbal expression. I merely extended them to caricature form. For example, for a depressed person, I had him kneel in an awkward off-balance position, head looking up, shoulder bowed as if to beg for someone to rescue him and be his reason for living.

As time went on, these postures suggested ways of sculpting interaction, including distances apart and up and down. I was also enabled to see how people give out two messages simultaneously such as, "Come here," and "go away." I came to call this kind of thing *family sculpture*. My use of it continues to evolve; it has turned out to be a powerful tool for creating awareness.

My going to Esalen in 1964 opened up a whole new dimension for me when I discovered what can be loosely referred to as the affective domain. Here I met people who had made lifelong studies, part of which I had observed but which others had carried much farther. They all concerned themselves with understanding and bettering the human condition, which was my absorbing interest as well. There were people such as Fritz Perls and his Gestalt Therapy, Eric Berne and his Transactional Analysis, Al Lowen's Bioenergetics, Charlotte Selver and Bernie Gunther in body awareness, Don Hayakawa with general semantics, and George Prince and Synectics. I was introduced to hypnotism, EST, LSD, parapsychology, sleep research, altered states of consciousness, marathons, nude and clothed massage and body image work, astrology, psychic healing and finally to yoga and Alan

Watts and Eastern ways of thought. This was a rich diet to digest. I ran it all through my three-layered hopper: What does this say about being human? What does it say about people becoming dysfunctional? What does it say about how growth can be rechanneled? I found that each of these persuasions had things to offer me, which in turn I could offer families.

The idea of self-esteem has always been central in my work. It now seems to me that self-esteem is as much related to the soul and spirit—the divine part of ourselves—as it is to our body, our emotions, our intellect and our I-Thou experiences, as well as our beliefs.

It further seems clear to me that whenever we start to try to help another human being, we must necessarily conclude with a deep appreciation of the human soul. Twenty years ago I was very careful to avoid references to, or even looking at, the soul because that was in the realm of organized religion and had no place in the "science" of psychotherapy.

Now I think perhaps that if religion had really worked, psychiatry may never have been born. I now see the human soul manifesting itself differently. For me, the feeling of the soul is reflected in how we value ourselves as human beings, how we treat our bodies and our emotions and the animal and plant life around us. Nurturing is a word that occurs very frequently in my thinking. That is not the same as being dependent or indulging oneself, but rather means a freedom to truly love and value oneself. I doubt whether a really nurtured self can ever abuse that self or inflict abuse on others. Furthermore, I believe that the human soul is really a manifestation of a life force or energy that goes on forming and reforming itself.

I believe that we are at the threshold of a breakthrough in tuning into a whole new world of the spirit. I find that people who achieve their sense of self-worth and self-value do not need to "freeload" on other people. They are clear that their survival is much more based on their ability to clearly know that they are their own total decision makers because they manage their own reactions and initiations. They believe in their bones that life is an evolving process, always capable of change. And they develop the courage to take risks. I think now that the therapist's job is to help this to come about. I see now about how to change the system so that it works toward developing this end rather than against it.

As I have been evolving, I have had experiences that tell me that there exists something that could be called the life force or universal mind. I know that there are many dimensions in this force that are powerful shapers in human behavior. It seems to me a little like the presence of electricity. It was always there, yet it waited for someone to identify it, then learn ways to use it for beneficial purposes. This probably could be referred to as psychic power, something all of us have experienced as atmosphere. There are already some ideas that each body is like an individual electrical generating unit. Our energy creator, and the amount and use of its own electrical power, is controlled mainly by belief and feelings of self-worth. I know that when I am in a state of low self-esteem, my energy is low and frequently misdirected—mostly against myself. For me, these experiences provide a very fruitful direction in which to go. In fact, I don't think I can help myself because so much is coming up that I am compelled to look at and investigate in this direction.

Now, let us return to another "growing edge," which is an interesting aspect and one that offers an important key in making an analogy between the family system and our institutional families. This is the fact that I see the same phenomena cropping up in organizational, social and governmental systems that I have seen in the family. My work with families, which I see as a microcosm of all human systems, prepared me well for the work I am now doing with larger systems.

Some fledgling concepts are beginning to emerge. Once the analogy has been made, it is not hard to see the similarity of family roles to institutional ones. Parent and child roles are similar to those of the president and his cabinet; marital roles are similar to those of Congress and the president. As a matter of fact, almost any group can find these analogies. If the parent acts as a boss, the system is likely to operate as a punishment-reward system. He and his "marital partner" are apt to be competitive or symbiotic, and the "children" have to be slaves, or competing or conniving to get recognition. Everyone suffers. Doesn't it sound familiar?

On the other hand, if the parent is a leader, he is likely to have "children" who relate with competency and creativeness and can be with a "mate" who truly shares. Try this on for size in a school system, a business, a church or any other governmental unit.

I have had the opportunity of working with a whole province, a whole hospital, a whole school system. There are unique opportunities and problems in them that I feel could be better understood, and therefore creatively changed, because I understood something about systems. For instance, no system remains open without a planned-for watcher from the outside—not as a policeman, but rather as someone in the radar tower helping planes land. It seems that without the outside input, the people in the system acclimatize themselves to the status quo and it slowly pervades the system in such a way that it loses each challenge, ceases to collect fresh, up-to-date information and, in general, just feeds itself by what is taken for granted. Death of one of the members or someone's leaving or entering may shake it up. If there is no new input, the slack of someone leaving or the budget created by a new member coming in may be momentarily chaotic, but then will settle down to the same old way, the same old cog-in-the-wheel syndrome.

As a family therapist, now I see the relatedness to what I do as potentially able to foster evolvement of each self in the family, and to create nurturing interrelationships in the family, in the institutions and generally in the world.

Obviously this is much more than technique. I didn't go too far in treatment of families and training before I found that I—as therapist or teacher—was a critical factor in how well I could teach people to begin the risk of change, and develop the reliable trust that went with that.

Therefore, my own continuing direction for myself is to look into, and experience, all of the things I find that could open up new vistas. And in just that way I feel my "growing edge" will continue to grow as these vistas open up before me.

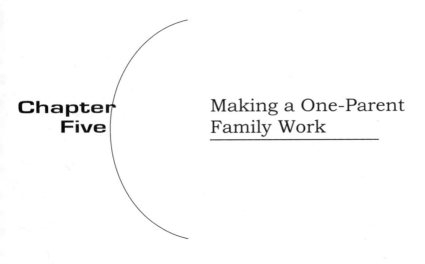

Chapter Five

Making a One-Parent Family Work

Introduction by Gloria Taylor

It is impossible to know when this article was written. It was no doubt put together at a time when the divorce and separation rate was much less than it is now. Regardless, Satir's recommendations are as valid now as then.

She begins by pointing out that the family unit consists of two parents who marry in their twenties and remain that way until they die. Second-rate families, in the prevailing views of the day, would be single parent, blended, and other non-traditional family units. The changes in attitude from then till now are for the reader to evaluate.

Satir's belief, ahead of her time, was that any family form could work well. Any unit that supports a healthy integrated child to grow to be an integrated adult with a rewarding life is one that works. As she puts it in this article, "It is not the form of the family that determines how well it works; rather, it is the relationships among the family members that make the difference." Satir wrote that she was seeing many new forms of family unit, where an adult male or female who is legally or blood-related is rearing those children alone. As she pointed out, it was estimated that one third of the children were living in one-parent or blended families and that the numbers seemed to be rising. Today she would look back on her paper and rightfully see herself as prophetic! Nor would she be surprised to hear that Canada has brought gay marriage into law.

As Satir insists, these new forms of family can work. She refers to the one-parent family but her words apply to any number of new forms. She stresses the theme of relationship when she writes , "the quality of the relationships within any family form determines, to a degree, how well that family works".

Satir talks about the intellectual, emotional, physical and spiritual development of the child. She defines the mature parent as an integrated being with high self-esteem who will help the child develop in such a way as to be able to rely on his/her own inner wisdom. All of this is challenging for adults who are in the position of having to guide and teach what they themselves have not yet mastered. Understanding this, she created Avanta, the Virginia Satir Network as a vehicle for training Satir methods to others who would continue the trainings internationally. She wrote and co-authored several books and many of her workshops were video-taped and are available today.

While acknowledging the possible fears and resentments that may reside in the hearts of single parents, she gently urges that people seek help for themselves as raising a child congruently can be more than a person feels he can handle on his own.

Addressing the need for children to have contact with the non-custodial parent, she stresses that this freedom be accorded the children. Then, as now, it was common to blame the other partner for everything and to run that through the children. Now we coach parents not to triangulate the children into the grief and resentments that belong with the parents and not with the children. If Satir were writing this today, she would include how to make children part of the process i.e. sharing with them as opposed to making decisions about and for them.

In a gentle sort of way, Virginia encourages people to grieve the loss of the relationships and the dreams of their futures. Rebuilding a life depends on this and she urges people to find kind listeners, friends, others in the same situation and to have fun. Fun was a feature of Virginia's perspective! As she reminds the reader a few pages later, "I recommend that you and your children develop strong senses of humor."

Satir gives permission for feelings, chaos and fears and then goes on to offer significant useful suggestions about the process of change. Her writings here are as meaningful today as when she first wrote them.

■ ■ ■

Many people still believe that the only family unit that can work well is one in which the parents marry and conceive their children in their 20's and stay married until their deaths, thus allowing for the children to have all of their care from the same adults. For centuries now this has been considered to be the only first-rate form for the family. All other forms (single-parent families, blended families, extended families with no blood ties and other non-traditional family units) still have a second-rate status in the eyes of many people.

I believe, however, that any family form can work well. My definition of working well is that the children grow up to be well-integrated adults, and that the adult or adults in charge also live rewarding lives. I have seen beautiful, healthy children and fulfilled adults present in every family form. I have also seen unhealthy children and unhealthy adults in every form. It is not the form of the family that determines how well it works; rather, it is the relationships among the family members that make the difference.

The concept that any family form can work is an important one in today's world. We are seeing the development of many new forms of the family, particularly in the Western world. One of the most prevalent new forms is the single-parent family, where an adult male or female who is related legally or by blood to a child or children, is rearing those children alone. We are also seeing many blended families, where the adults in the family are not the ones who together conceived the children; rather, the family has been created from divorce and remarriage or adoption. In fact, it is estimated that at this time roughly one-third of all of our children live in either blended families or one-parent families, and that number seems to be rising. With so many children being raised in new family forms, it is very important that we remember that such forms can work well.

In this writing, I will direct my thoughts to the one-parent family. I will not consider the reasons for the development of this form; rather, I will talk about the form as it exists, and share ideas about how it can be first-rate. This big question is: "How can things be managed in such a way that everybody wins?" This is the theme of this chapter.

I am especially directing my discourse to those persons who felt a reasonable certainty at the time of the conception of their child that two parents would be together during the maturing years of that child. I also believe that much of what I write here will be applicable to any person who is in the position of raising a child alone. I leave it to the reader to use the parts that they feel fit for them.

The therapist or human educator who reads this can find creative ways to communicate to clients some of the points I highlight here. This can be rewarding to both the therapist and the family involved. It is important to remember that the one-parent family can work and work well; the challenge is in finding ways to make it happen.

As I said before, the quality of the relationships within any family form determine, to a great degree, how well that family works. All families share this common denominator: One of the keys to relationships working well is the degree of self-worth felt by each family member.

A person with high self-worth is able to make sense of what is going on around him. She can become self-reliant. He becomes confident in himself. She is able to be intimate with others and has meaningful relationships with both males and females.

The main concern in one-parent families is how to care for the maturing child or children. So it helps to know about children and maturation. A child is a new being who requires the help of others to obtain maturation. Maturation has many aspects. Following are the bare bones of it.

The child has physical needs. The child needs the proper physical care so that she or he can grow up healthy and strong. The child also needs knowledge about how to physically care for himself or herself.

The child's intellectual development requires mental stimulation, both a formal and informal education, to deepen the mind and make it versatile and effective.

The child has emotional needs. The emotional part requires that the child learn how to acknowledge, direct, and utilize feelings for his or her own health and enriched self.

The child has socialization needs. The social experience requires a child to learn how to enrich his or her life with others, to build meaningful relationships with person of both sexes, and to enter into ways of cooperating and building with others.

He or she has sensual needs. The development of the sensual self requires that the child learn how to use his or her senses to experience the variety of life: the song, the dance, the fragrances, the colors, and the textures of the world.

The child has spiritual needs. The spiritual aspect requires that the child experience his or her life force, and understand that we are all connected with a universal life force.

The parents need to help the child develop and integrate each of these aspects so that maturation is a process resulting in an integrated human being with a high sense of self-esteem. The child also needs help to develop her or his ability to find and rely on his or her own inner wisdom.

Helping a child mature in all of these aspects is a tall order for any adult who brings up children. It is especially challenging for adults who have not yet completed total maturation for themselves. When this is the case, the adults are in the position of having to teach and guide what they have not yet mastered themselves. If you sense that this is your situation, I recommend that you find and access places and people to learn what you need, whether family members, change groups, or professional counseling. Adults in every family form are faced with this challenge. However, it shows up more clearly when one is faced with making a one-parent family work.

Some people feel that seeking help in their own maturation process is somehow shameful. There need be no shame. If there is a gap between what you would like to do as a parent and what you are actually able to do, it is wise to seek help. This kind of gap often brings up a lot of fear, frustration and resentment. Unknowingly, this can become centered on the children and be perceived as a child problem rather than an adult problem. It's very important to determine what kinds of problems exist, and to own the ones that you are helping to create.

A child also needs to grow toward having a loving, accepting view of his or her own sex, and placing an equal value on persons of the other sex. Children reflect the values of their parents. The parent who has come to value himself or herself, and to value the other sex, will help her/his children value their own and the other sex.

In order to accomplish this, the head of the one-parent family needs first to hold or acquire those values. Then, he or she will look for opportunities to have male and female adult friends present and encourage the sons and daughters to do the same. There is no teaching greater than the teaching of modeling.

Every child knows, on a deep level, how his or her parent feels about his or her own sex and about the other sex. Out of loyalty to that parent, the child will often assume the parent's values for herself or himself.

No man really knows what it is like to be a girl or a woman, and no woman truly knows what it is really like to be a boy or a man. Growing boys need to have both trusted adult male and female guides. Growing girls need both too. The managing adult consciously needs to look for and encourage the presence of such guides in the child's life. Such adults may be within the family: grandparents, aunts or uncles, older cousins, close friends, the other parent, for example. If your family does not provide such guides, you can seek them elsewhere in boys' clubs and girls' clubs, in church, among the good teachers at your child's school. The main point is to recognize your child's needs for trusted adult companions of both sexes, and then to make certain they have contact with such people.

The age of the child at the departure of one of the parents has a bearing on the situation. Speaking from the child's point of view, there always were, and still are, two parents, even if one has left or died. If one parent is not physically present, he or she is present in the fantasy of the child. This is part of the inner life of the child.

As I have explained in the section on co-parenting, it is important, if possible, that the child have contact with the departed parent. In that way, the child can form, instead of fantasies, real pictures of that parent. If it is not possible for the child to have contact with that parent, then the managing parent will want to be as factual as possible when talking with the child about the absent parent.

Repression of the child's fantasies sometimes occurs in some living climates within households. When grief over the departed parent is unresolved, or where anger about the departure has not been handled, repression is more likely. Of course, when any of our dreams come to an end, there is always sadness and disappointment. Allowing yourself and your children to successfully mourn will help to ensure that repression isn't necessary in your home.

In the case of divorce, I think it is extremely important for the child to have equal access to both parents. There are many reasons for this. One of the big ones is to find as many resources as possible to help in the raising of the growing child. The other parent is one very important resource.

It is often hard for either or both parents to give to their children freedom of access to the other parent. This is especially true when the breaking up of the parent's original dream has become particularly unpleasant, or when there has been a large load of blame in the process of the parting. In time, however, it is important that this freedom be accorded the child.

For many years, our society and our courts have created an adversarial situation in the case of divorce. The result of this has been to make one parent "wrong" and one parent "right." The children, traditionally, have been placed with the "right" parent (usually the mother), and the "wrong" parent (usually the father) has only limited visiting privileges. Now, more and more people are realizing that while spouses divorce, parents do not divorce their children. They are seeing that one of the most destructive things about divorce for the child is the virtual loss of one parent. Now, people realize that a child needs both an active mother and an active father.

Divorced parents can work together in helpful ways so that children can grow well. This is most possible after the parents have "cleared the decks" regarding the breaking up of their mutual dream, and have put their blaming and guilt feelings behind them.

Another big thing is that it is important for children to have real pictures of each of their parents. This is most easily accomplished when the child has equal contact with each parent. The parents, as well as the children, can benefit from this kind of situation. It has been my experience that, when divorced parents decide they must find ways to continue to work together in the interest of their children, the parents often discover in themselves things they never knew existed. I've also had many divorced parents tell me that, through working together in the interest of their mutual children, they have become better friends.

Regardless of the reason for the loss of one parent, it is important for all family members, children as well as adult, to freely mourn that loss. Mourning involves allowing yourself to fully experience the loss, your feelings about it, and the pain attached to it. By successfully going through this tender and painful period, you can become open to the new possibilities that will emerge.

If you try to go on with life without mourning your loss, your "decks are not cleared" for your new life to begin. The shaping of a satisfying, rewarding new life depends upon your being emotionally free to fully mourn the loss of your old dream, and your partner in that dream.

The mourning process, listed in steps, goes something like this. First, you develop an awareness that life presents situations over which you have no control. Whether those situations seem right or wrong is not the issue.

If one of the divorced spouses remarries, this is another phase to be coped with. Strong feelings may emerge for the other parent, and he or she needs to acknowledge, express, and own those feelings. There may be difficulties in integrating that new marriage partner into the family. However, this is also a chance for the child to have more loving adults in his or her life. The chances are that if the one-parent family has been working well, the inclusion of a new mate for either spouse will be easier to integrate. (That, of course, is the subject for another paper.)

Third, you need own your own feelings. Examples of ownership are: "I am so angry!" and "I feel so bad." I feel so helpless." Often, however, people get stuck in blaming another person for their feelings. Examples of blame feelings are: "You make me feel so angry! You make me feel so bad." Sometimes blame feelings come out like this: "Why did you do this or that to me?" or "Why does it happen to me?"

It is important that you know the difference between feelings that you own as yours and your blame of yourself and others. As long as you blame others for your situation or your pain, it will be difficult for you to create a hopeful, joyful new life for yourself.

If your blame feelings dominate, or if you feel stuck in them, it will be valuable to seek professional help because you are stifling your own growth. You are putting your energy into non-growthful places. You are also seriously threatening your children's growth, especially if they are young. For your happiness and for the wise guidance of your children, you need to move through this tender and painful period.

Fourth, you need to be forgiving of yourself for whatever feelings come out. They are you, of course, but they are also an emerging part of you. Letting your feelings come out begins the process of integrating for the new life that has to follow. In the long run, these feelings are only temporary ones. However, it is necessary for you, and for your children, that they be expressed.

Part of the mourning process is to experience your feelings toward the departed one. That means giving expression to the pains and the angers, as well as the valuable parts and the love.

It helps to remember during this period that we are all human beings with "good" parts and "bad" ones. There are few documented cases of human saints (all "good") or human devils (all "bad"). You are a combination of these qualities, as is your lost one. If you find yourself concentrating on only the saintly qualities or only the devil-like qualities of your lost one, you are remembering a stereotype of a person, not the total human being.

If it fits for you, find a trusted person with whom you can share the expressions of your feelings around this period. It often helps to have support. You have been injured, and injury requires that you allow yourself to feel it so that you can heal yourself.

In the long run, these mourning feelings are only temporary ones. It can be difficult to give them expression, especially if they are of the so-called "negative" type such as anger and sorrow for example. Most human beings resist going into something new. The resistance is even greater when it is accompanied by a deep feeling of loss and pain. However, it is necessary to mourn if you are to rebuild. It is necessary to encourage your children to do the same. If it is truly difficult for you, find people to support you though this process.

It is also important to know that this process does not happen all at once. When we are in the middle of something painful, it is hard to see outside of it. Be patient with yourself.

Also, when we experience very strong feelings, often our minds don't work very well. We might find ourselves reacting as we reacted before the loss occurred. I still hear people talk of reaching for the hand of a lost one who has died. Others tell me that, weeks and months after the loss, they find themselves anticipating the entry of the lost one at a certain time of day. We have to give ourselves time to adjust to a new situation.

While this process is difficult, it is also rewarding and productive. It will allow you to shape a satisfying new life. Your new life will be different, and it can be very rewarding and fulfilling. Believe that. Believe in your abilities and resources. Believe in your wisdom as you proceed through the steps of mourning. When you have successfully passed through this phase, you will experience a new integration of yourself. New thoughts of hope and images of possibilities will begin to emerge.

How well you cope with the realities and demands of becoming the head of a single-parent household will have something to do with the degree of self-esteem you have already developed, and with the freedom you feel to be in touch with your feelings.

Because we are human, we need to find explanations for things that happen. When faced with a loss, two possible explanations people may create are: (1) "Poor Me" (blaming oneself) or (2) "It's all his/her fault" (blaming another). Blaming oneself is a version of "I am nothing," and creates guilt. Blaming the other is simply a reverse of blame of self. Both impede your ability to construct your new life, and both have negative lessons for your children.

Here is an example of how such coping postures affect children. Say a woman is the head of a single-parent family. She blames herself or her former partner. Her children will learn both explicit and implicit lessons from their mother, and they, in turn, will reflect that learning in their own behavior and attitude.

The woman's daughter might, for example, learn things like, "Never trust a man," or "You must always do what a man wants in order to please him." These kinds of teachings come back to haunt the individual. Neither of the teachings will help the daughter to have a positive view of herself or of men.

The woman's son may learn that "Don't be like your father." Since the son is a boy, it may be understood by him that to be a male is bad. A further, and even more erosive, response is to entwine her son so closely with herself that he cannot feel comfortable with other women.

These are extremes. However, they exist all too frequently.

If the single parent is male, he can fall into the same traps by blaming himself or his former wife. Similar results may occur for his sons and daughters. Many variations on these kinds of learnings exist when the loss of a partner is treated mainly from a blame standpoint.

I think it is very helpful to develop a support group for yourself, and particularly to include in that group other single parents. It helps to keep in your consciousness people who are also heading one-parent families. Such people can share with you the agonies and joys of their experience, their successes and failures, as well as practical how-to advice.

It is important to have friends, to have fun, and to do things that you especially enjoy with other adults. If all you do is work and parent, then life gets very bleak. This, of course, reflects on your children. You need to have time for yourself and the stimulation that pursuing interests and having companionship from other adults can bring.

It is also helpful to remember that your mental health and outlook on life have a lot to do with feeling satisfied and gratified in your life. Supportive friends, interests outside of the home, and time to yourself can help you maintain a positive attitude, a healthy outlook on life, and a high sense of self-esteem.

One of the big challenges for the single parent is to develop a fulfilling life. Unfulfilled parents make greater difficulties for children. There are some general hints that can help make a single-parent family work well.

First, allow yourself and your children to go through a mourning period following the loss of one parent whether that loss is by death, departures or divorce.

Second, the facts and feelings surrounding a family becoming a one-parent family are two very different things. For a healthy one-parent family, I would recommend that the children know the real facts from all the people concerned, not just bias from one parent. Children need to know these facts as fully as they are known by the adults. It helps, too, if they are told about the facts as they are occurring, if possible. If not then, the children should know about them as soon as possible. Children are never too young to be told these facts, nor are they ever too old.

Children sense, even more than their parents perhaps, what is going on. If they are not told the facts, they make up their own version of them. They often do this to the detriment of their own self-worth. They may, for example, blame themselves if their parents divorce. Another result is that children often will bottle things up inside themselves, which can cause needless anguish, illness, and emotional pain.

Third, be very careful not to use your children against the other parent or to use that parent against your children. If this goes on, it will show up in the form of damaged relationships in the family. The communication is such that the child cannot state what is going on. He or she will have to internalize it; this is where a lot of troubles come from.

Fourth, the needs of the children cannot wait. After the departure of one parent, through death or divorce or other reasons, life must go on. There must be food and shelter. Bills must be paid. Life must be reordered and reprioritized. This requires planning and making decisions at a time when it may be difficult to plan and decide.

It may be helpful in the business of reordering to find a friend or support group to provide advice, information, and friendship. There are even special counseling centers in some colleges, YMCAs and local agencies that exist to help people in transition make these kinds of decisions. If you sense it would fit for you, seek out this kind of help.

All of these tasks will be easier, of course, if the parent in charge is already skillful in these areas and if the family members have already learned to work well together. If this is not your situation, find resources to help you with these jobs.

Fifth, I recommend that you and your children develop strong senses of humor. Humor cures many things, and can be invaluable during a difficult period of your life.

Sixth, if possible, set up a mutual learning and teaching situation with your children. I have so often been impressed with the enormous resources of children. They have a great deal to offer any parent, and can be especially helpful in a single-parent situation. If you are all tied up with the idea that to be a parent means that one has to be all things to all people, and to know everything, there is no opportunity for you to seek and develop the resources of your children.

Seventh, another thing to become aware of is that your children are asking for leadership. This is leadership instead of bossing. You must remember that every member of your family, no matter how young or old, has something worthwhile to contribute. Make it your business to find it and to cultivate it.

It's also important to remember that yes and no can be expressions of boundaries and possibilities. Saying yes or no to your children does not determine who is loved by you and who is rejected. To do fulfilling yeses and noes, it is important to be as fully informed about the request as possible. If you don't have the information you need, it is better to say, "I can't do that now," or "Let's wait" rather than to give a yes or no that is not fully there.

When the time comes that an initially participating parent leaves, there is usually a mixture of feelings: shock, bewilderment, anger, helplessness, frustration and sometimes relief. These feelings are part of the often difficult reality that confronts single parents. They, as well as other practical considerations, will require a creative struggle. However, it helps to remember that struggling is probably not a new experience for you or your children. All of us need to learn to struggle creatively. It is this kind of coping that gives our lives texture.

It is also helpful to be aware that we are all human beings, doing human things, and that most of us are doing the best we can. Because we live in a world that has stresses and threats as well as opportunities, we sometimes are not able to see that clearly. And sometimes, when one parent departs, the threats and stresses are so overwhelming that it is easy to feel that everything is too much to cope with. In this state, it can be hard to feel hopeful and to search out the opportunities we need to give us hope.

In those dark times, keep in your awareness that you are a miracle. All human beings are miracles. What other living form has the potentials and possibilities as the human being? Sometimes we forget how rich we are in our resources. When we forget, we get depressed, ill and hopeless. Yet, it doesn't have to be that way. There are other ways.

If we can hold on to our high sense of self-worth, our willingness to risk, our understanding that birth and death, as well as death and rebirth, are part of the human package, life does have endless possibilities. Life can be viewed a little like a bas-relief. As one thing has been passed, another thing begins to emerge. Keeping in mind the possibility that there is hope for a rich new life following a loss can enable you to really look for and find the resources that you need.

You have many places to look for resources. You have personal abilities and skills. You can look at your degree of personal integration (and build upon it). You can look at and learn from your experience. Throughout this process, you may have newly awakened creative abilities.

You can keep these in mind, and at hand, as you pay attention to the practical matters of being a single parent (your finances, living arrangements, the reshaping of your context) so you can see what needs to be done.

Facing a new situation takes all of us into the unknown. That can seem scary, especially when it is as a result of the breaking up of a dream and the loss of a marriage partner.

Such losses are not pleasant. I do, however, feel that they are part of life and that none of us is ever in a position to predict. If we can get all the "Ain't it Awful's" and "Poor Me's" out of the way, we can become creative. We can free our energy for other parts of ourselves to grow and become fulfilled. Life goes on like a river, always turning up new possibilities if we are open to them.

As the head of a single-parent family, you are not one of society's rejects. You are one of society's creative possibilities. Hold on to that thought.

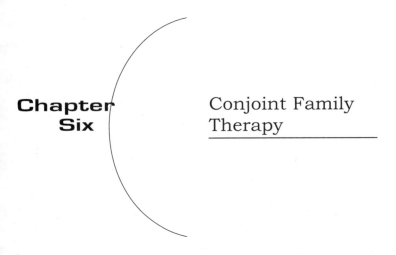

Chapter Six

Conjoint Family Therapy

Introduction by Stephen Smith

In 1993, while I was working at an addictions treatment center, I began to study the work of Virginia Satir. That study, which continues to the present, transformed the way I look at the therapeutic enterprise. Much of the theory and method that brought about that transformation is included in this chapter. Satir elucidates many elements of her theory and method of family therapy, which she developed while working with Gregory Bateson, Jay Haley, John Weakland and Don D. Jackson at the Mental Research Institute. She proposes that the focus of intervention be on the relationships between parts of the family system rather than the parts themselves.

There are two very important implications of this approach. First, Satir draws attention away from individual parts as the carriers of system problems and in this way removes blame from the individual as responsible for the pathology represented by symptoms. The identified problem is not the problem; the way the system copes with the problem is the problem. Satir considers that the symptom was merely a visible sign of systemic problems that result from the suppression of questions and therefore the suppression of clear, non-ambiguous communication. Second, treating the symptom without changing the system in which it arose will merely result in repetition of the symptom in the same or another form. Her therapy is not intended to be corrective in terms of the symptom, but growth oriented in terms of the whole system.

Satir goes on to describe what a healthy individual looks like in terms of congruence, high self-esteem, awareness of himself/ herself as a choice maker, and responsible for the outcomes of such choices. This description is carried over in her portrayal of a competent therapist. Her implication is that the therapist becomes part of the system during an intervention, and if the therapist is not capable of clear, unambiguous communication, change for the better will not come about as the family will respond in its usual dysfunction pattern.

The Satir model of therapy transforms the role of the therapist from adjudicator of right and wrong to explorer in terms of asking the questions the participants have suppressed. It is the expression of these questions that leads to the elucidation of the rules that prevent clear communication between participants. As the therapist exposes the hidden rules under which families often operate, participants can now make choices about which rules they wish to keep and those they wish to discard because they no longer fit.

In this chapter, Satir clearly demonstrates how her beliefs about people and the therapeutic process directly inform her practice. She provides an opportunity for any therapist willing to study her model to develop a method of practice that creates an atmosphere of trust and respect that is conducive to real change.

■ ■ ■

My therapy centers around the application of concepts of interaction. The therapy deals directly with the present rules and processes of individuals by exploring their family system. An overlapping network of examination occurs as the therapy uncovers family rules and processes. I see the family as an operating unit with rules for its maintenance, and all the individuals within this unit as functioning with uniqueness. This unit is a system with rules related to precedence, too, so that when separate rules conflict with family rules, there is an awareness of what will happen next.

I see behavior as the result of interactions. Appropriate behavior occurs as individual members fulfill their particular role contract in the context of the continually changing situation. Appropriate behavior furthers enjoyment and development of self, as well as furthering the common goals of the family. Inappropriate behavior signals dysfunction. I see a symptom as a report. The child in trouble reports that the marital unit functions with some discrepancy. His symptoms distort, but make obvious, his experience of inhibiting communication.

Communication is the means by which needs are met. A human being cannot get his needs met if he cannot communicate. Within the family system one learns how or how not to communicate. Families who deal with a created or invented reality, who deny what seems to be objectivity, will produce members who report this by their symptoms. Often I find that dysfunctional families use direct questions infrequently. They hint rather than speak to each other, or they prefer to suppress questions. I see anxiety, hostility and finally helplessness as the outcome of a family process that suppresses questions. Suppose that now I were speaking rather than writing, and that you had to report what I say. If you miss something, if you do not understand, and you cannot ask questions, you become anxious. If you miss hearing to any significant degree, you become hostile. If you continue missing, you will finally become helpless.

Of course, questions are risks. If families fear being exposed by questions, they forbid or dilute this risk. Families in which self-esteem is low frequently do this. I believe that if the two architects, the male and the female who got together sexually to begin the family, have high self-esteem, their building will produce a system in which all members value self. All members in this kind of system can speak of and can raise questions about what they individually perceive as reality. All members, as well as the family unit itself, will make and use flexible, appropriate, satisfying and subject-to-change rules. This family unit will form a link to society that is open and hopeful.

One of the main emphases in my therapy is that of strengthening self-esteem. I am a positive person, who believes that people try to do the best they can with what they know. I see my work as having two main parts, learning and experience. I teach each person, relating to him through his uniqueness, by allowing and encouraging him to experience. Family members need to experience self and each other. I use talk, clear communication which at times sounds simplistic and repetitious, in my search for the thing being explicitly communicated to me. I use exercises and games that I have developed to speed up and intensify the experience of family communication. These exercises and games rely on the human imagination and the human senses. I work to deepen awareness and to intensify appreciation for communication. Looking, listening, paying attention, getting understanding, and making meaning are all part of this. Most of my structured experiences show the importance our bodies have in communication. I don't believe a person who is saying one thing and whose body contradicts him. I think a person is leveling with me when all of him is congruent. His body, his focus, his movement, his words, his tone, his facial muscles—when all come to me on one level—then I can hear what a person says. I am able to experience him clearly, and I can believe him.

The purpose and the methods of my therapy allow persons to know that they can communicate. They can be safe because they can be known by others, and they can know others. In therapy I work to help them realize that the outcome of communication, or what actually happens, depends upon themselves. Whether or not a family is a good place to be and to live, and to enjoy, depends on the knowing and the being known. The appreciation of the knowing and the being known causes family members to be conscious of value. They value themselves and each other, building self-esteem. They respect self and others enough to choose to be clear. They communicate clearly to show self and others who they are, and where they are. They can trust because of the openness. The unit that this kind of family makes is a good place to be.

Theoretical Foundation of Therapy

The main premise underlying the idea that symptoms are a family production is the notion that all families operate as systems. I see symptoms within individuals as embodiments of family dysfunction within the family system. Therapy for the total family unit is logical.

Family systems seem to have order and sequence, and they seem to be reliable. Family members, often unconsciously, know what will happen next. Family systems also appear to be disproportionate. We all have the need to grow in many areas, such as physical, emotional, social, and intellectual; in terms of survival, intimacy, productivity, and making sense and order. These growth needs are rarely met, and are not met equally for all the individuals within a family. The system may meet the needs of some members partially, and some may be left out altogether.

The system has order and sequence itself that has decision-making processes, and rules for negotiation and power. Rules of the system control communication: who speaks, who speaks for whom, who speaks attributing blame or credit to another. All are observable factors of a family system.

From this point of view, the behavior of any family member is entirely appropriate and understandable. Member behavior is appropriate in terms of the family's own system. The behavior of an individual may not fit his own growth needs, nor seem to suit the expectations of other family members, but it does suit the family system. Understanding the system, then, allows understanding of the symptom bearer or the identified patient.

This approach began as I observed that families with a schizophrenic child reported that things between the marital pair were pretty perfect. Their crazy son or daughter made life a problem for them. Evidences of personal inadequacies, frustrations and disappointments in the marital relationship were covered up. As the sick child got better, the husband-wife relationship got worse. The pathology was in the unit rather than in the individual.

Studying communication patterns of these families led to the *double-bind theory*. Simply stated, the double-bind theory asserts that the schizophrenic child learns behavior and communication within a situation of simultaneous contradiction. The child receives one message verbally, another non-verbally. For example, a mother may say, "Come close to Mother, Johnny, if you love her," while at that moment expressing rigidity through her gestures.

Now we cannot not respond. So if we receive double messages from a survival figure, we are bound into a situation in which meaning, responses—the "shoulds" that we depend on—and expectations assault growth. Children in situations of this sort develop symptoms. But the point is not that inadequate parents produce sick children. The point is that bizarre, seemingly meaningless behavior from symptom bearers is appropriate behavior until the situation of the family or the universe of the symptom bearer is changed. The communication patterns of continual assault must be changed. In my opinion, these communication patterns are outside a family's awareness. Theoretically, the first step in therapy is to bring these patterns of the family into their awareness.

Early work comparing different kinds of families—families with delinquent members, under-achievers, or individuals with ulcerative colitis, for example—indicates that different kinds of dysfunctional systems lead to different sorts of symptoms. What kind of family develops depends upon the male and the female, the architects, of the family, and upon the families of *their* previous lives. Clinically and impressionistically it appears that the system a family develops begins in the courtship of the male and the female, and develops and is modified as the marriage goes along, integrating children into the family. The important things, however, seem to lie not so much in the obvious. When one is trying to find out the meaning of present behavior, one must uncover the network of rules that the family communication utilizes. What are the rules now? Who may do what? Under what conditions? Who may comment, and on what may he comment?

I have found that families with symptom bearers characteristically have rules that do not clearly allow for recognition of the uniqueness and separateness of each person in the family. First names tend not to be used; members do not look at each other when speaking. Decisions seem to occur as a power struggle rather than as a negotiable process recognizing objective reality. Rules tend to suppress difference; difference seems representative of criticism to family members. In these families, the needs that all human beings have to survive, grow, get close to others, and produce are fulfilled—and often distorted—within conflict. The symptoms of these members comment upon the discrepancy between their own growth needs and the rules of the situation they must depend upon.

Growth is a struggle, and I see each child as struggling to find his own power in a situation where there already are powerful persons who may not value nor help his personal efforts for power. Each child struggles for independence, but he lives within a situation of interdependency. He wishes to be a sexual person, but he may find a confusion of secrecy hiding genital differences. As a child who produces, he may find that his worth is measured primarily by his production. He sees, hears, feels and thinks. But may he share his perceptions without anyone "dropping dead"; that is, without anyone manifesting pain or anger implying death or destruction?

I assume that symptoms signify frustration of growth. These can be looked at three ways. First, who labeled what behavior as a symptom, or what actual behavior is being called a symptom by whom? Second, what does the symptom say about growth frustration for the person bearing the symptom? Finally, how does this growth frustration maintain survival for the family and maintain relationships? In other words, how does the symptom show the presence of pain, trouble or confusion in the family? Recognizing the symptom as appropriate behavior to an inappropriate system has therapeutic implication.

The family as one whole unit should be seen together in one time and in one place. Therapy begins by uncovering and under-standing the family's currently operating system. The growth needs of each member are seen as taking place in a context. Behavior, in contrast, is not seen as pathology of the individual, or as isolated, or as "afflicted". This shift makes each person's behavior become understandable, and further, it allows treatment emphasis to shift from "disease" to "growth."

After early exploration has centered around understanding, the operation of the current system—how each person is reacting to these rules—is uncovered. Then comes the job of changing the system, of education, re-education, and creating experiences of safe, clear communication while in the presence of the therapist. I frequently find in dysfunctional families that members do not ask simple fact-finding questions, nor expect clear answers. As the therapist gets each person to manifest himself clearly in a climate of safety, each person acquires the strength, the know-how, and actually the bravery to do this. As each family member learns to communicate, and does communicate, he is able to sat-isfy his needs more directly. As a family begins talking straight, without conflictual qualifications, the family's rules will begin to change. Changing the rules changes the system. A pathological atmosphere can become a healthy atmosphere.

Therapists are therefore concerned with process, more than with outcome. How meanings are sent, how they are received, no matter what the content, is the point. The therapist pays atten-tion to the processes that reveal the network of commitment and contract between family members. The therapist wants to ensure that what is meant is what is said and what is heard. The thera-pist wants to ensure that each person has esteem, for himself and from his family group.

Attitudes I Work From

Over the years I have developed a picture of what the human being, living humanly, is like. He is a person who understands, values, and develops his body, finding it beautiful and useful; a person who is real and honest to and about himself and others; a person who is willing to take risks, to be creative, to manifest competence; to change when the situation calls for it; and to find ways to accommodate to what is new and different, keeping that part of the old that is still useful and discarding what is not. With healthy human beings, feeling and communication are the same. As a matter of fact, when I see a person in whom feeling and communication are the same, I know the treatment is complete.

The healthy person can do without the hidden; he can see himself the way others see him; he can tell another what he hopes, fears, and expects. He can disagree, he can make choices, he can learn through practice. He accepts responsibility for his own thinking, his own hearing, and his own seeing. He knows himself. He deals with the actual world, not just his "wish."

As we become more healthy, we free ourselves from the harm of the past. We achieve a maturity. Seeing maturity as a good is a very important concept in my therapy. I think a mature person is in charge of himself. He can make choices; he has the judgment to know that his choices are his limits. He makes decisions on the basis of accurate perceptions about himself and others, and the context in which he finds himself. He acknowledges his choices; he owns his choices. Because his decisions are his own, he accepts responsibility for their outcome. Each of us, I think, bears the responsibility of being aware of what we give out to ask the other person to deal with. But at the same time, I have control over the choice of whether or not to act and the course of action I take. For this, I can be held responsible to myself as well as to others. I can not be responsible for what is presented to me, only for my response to it.

These interdependences make us conscious of the way we follow models. We are models for each other. We are responsible for being clear, congruent models.

This vital business that goes on in families is what I call *people-making.* Healthy families make healthy people. Dysfunctional families make unhealthy people. A family is a bit like a factory; the kind of factory determines the product. Good peoplemaking goes on where self-worth is high; communication is direct, clear, specific, and honest; rules are flexible, human, appropriate, and subject to change; and the link to society is open and hopeful.

It is my attitude that children in a family reflect the marital situation in which they are reared. Differences do exist. Father is a male and mother is a female. That is a big difference. If either father or mother sees difference of any sort as something to fear, or the source of conflict, then there is a war-like atmosphere with a hurtful, inhibiting set of family rules. On the other hand, if difference is seen as pleasant, as an opportunity to explore and to gain understanding, then the family blueprint is a peaceful one where growth, and fun and the good things of life can occur. I have found that a person's reaction to differences—and to differentness—is an index of his ability to adapt to growth and change. It also indicates what attitudes he will have toward other members of his family, and whether he will be able to express these attitudes directly or not.

Blueprints are made up of interdependences and the interactional transactions. The rules, who the models are, and what the messages about the desirability of growth are create a blueprint for each individual. He learns to evaluate, and to act on new experiences. He learns whether or not to be close to others. The family is the place where a human being finds out about himself. The family is the place where he first decides whether or not he is worthwhile. He first learns what other people are like. He learns how to relate to others and to the world. The family is the keeper of the essential learnings.

Now the teaching process includes the following: a clear idea of what is to be taught, an awareness that each parent has of what he is modeling, a knowledge of how to interest the other in following that model, and the communication to make it work. Families teach to a purpose in peoplemaking. Each person somehow, whether ideally or not, gets involved in the peoplemaking. Each person looks to the family for direction, freedom, encouragement, nurturance and appreciation for uniqueness.

Persons in an ideal family, to me, are people who clearly show their own uniqueness, who demonstrate their power, who clearly show their sexuality, who demonstrate their ability to share through understanding, kindness, and affection, who use their common sense, and who are realistic and responsible. That may sound like an impossibility, but it is my attitude that persons can try to keep moving in that direction while respecting where they are. The key words are unique, powerful, sexual, sharing, sensible, realistic and responsible.

The family is really the place where a person can learn and can develop into this ideal person. But the fact that each person at any single moment in a family is a whole person is a significant notion to grasp. No matter whether this human being is two weeks old, or 15, or 35, or 85 years old, he is a whole person. He has a right to expect peoplemaking from his family. The disappointment that a grown man experiences at losing a desired job is no more painful than that of a four-year old who loses his favorite toy. The experience of disappointment is the same at any age. The feeling in a child who is the brunt of a tirade from an angry mother is no different from the woman's feelings if she has been the brunt of the tirade of an angry husband, or vice versa.

Children seem to thrive on the knowledge that their world of hope, fear, mistakes, imperfections, and successes is a world also known and shared by their parents. Parents who choose authority, rather than honestly expressing feelings, seem phony to their children. If a child becomes distrustful of his parents, he extends the feelings into isolation and general feelings of unsureness and rebellion.

Now to get back to the key words. I think it isn't necessary to explain what I mean by "sensible," "sharing," and "realistic." I use those words the same way you do. When it comes to "uniqueness," "power," and "sexuality," I want to go into more depth. Understanding these concepts is important in the family blueprint.

I believe uniqueness is the key word to self-worth. We get together on the basis of our similarities, and we grow on the basis of our differences. We need both. It is this combination of sameness and differentness in a human being that I call *uniqueness*. Helping a child to value the difference between his parents becomes an important part of his learning. Appreciating himself is, too. If infants don't have the opportunity to be treated as unique from the beginning of their lives, it will become difficult for them to react as whole people. They will be handicapped.

Now about the key word, *power*. Body power develops first. The infant's first cry is most welcome. We greet physical coordination with joy. He is expected to grow and manage his body. I have noticed that parents will have endless patience teaching their child body power, showing joy at each successful effort. I think showing joy at each successful effort is a suitable way to teach the other areas of power, too. The other areas of power are intellectual, emotional, social, material, and spiritual. It is my attitude that if we use patience and respond to the expression of the child's newfound power with joy and approval, we are successful. Emotional power seems scariest, perhaps because adults may not trust their own emotional power.

Another area of difficulty is frequently found as the family teaches sex—in its broadest sense maleness and femaleness. What a child decides about this reflects not at all what parents say, but how they enjoy differences.

I've said a lot about teaching, but of course it's not possible to teach family members what to do in every situation. However, I have found that the family that has emphasized the self-worth of whole people will discover that these people know what to do, because they have developed judgment as they made their own individual choices all along.

Some of the How of Therapy

Experiencing and sharing what is for family members is the main part of my therapy. It begins as two persons look at each other. I want people to experience one another. Suppose you are face to face with me; your senses take in what I look like, how I sound, what I smell like, and if you happen to touch me, how I feel to you. Your brain then reports what this means to you, calling upon your past experiences, particularly with your parents and other authority figures, your book learning, and your ability to use this information to explain the message from your senses. Depending upon what your brain reports, you feel comfortable or uncomfortable; your body is loose or tight. And I am going through the same thing. My senses are taking in, I am in contact with my past experiences, my values and expectations. I feel my body reacting. It is doing something because you and I are looking at each other. But what our brains "know" about the other are guesses and fantasies, until we check out facts.

Let's say you and I are a man and a woman who are in one of the normal life crises. Our adult daughter, Linda, is moving to an apartment of her own. This particular crisis has a heavy sadness for most families. A child's leaving is a big loss. Now, as the man, I take you in. I feel pleasure in your presence, I see an unusual look of resignation about your face, your eyes look sad to me and so I guess that you do not approve of Linda's plan. If I am the woman, I take you in. You are the same contented person that I have felt comfortable with for 25 years, yet there is a clear evidence of concern, which looks like worry to me. I have a fantasy of you explaining to Linda how living in a city apartment can be expensive, lonely and possibly dangerous.

All this takes place in a fraction of a second, before either of us has said a word. When we begin to talk openly, freely, trustingly, we find our guesses and fantasies have changed. As the man, I hear you say that not only do you approve of Linda's independence, you envy her a little. You share your sadness in anticipating the natural loneliness that occurs when a child moves out. As the woman, I hear that you admire Linda's spirit. When I listen to you talk, you discuss judgment and choice, and you let me understand how you hope we have given her enough choices to help her develop judgment.

In consciously checking each other out, you and I have shared; we've become aware of each other. We are in a very real sense more visible to each other; we've become more accessible. We appreciate each other more as we become more aware. By verbally checking out sensory communication we get a fuller and more accurate dimension. And we can feel more secure when we are not guessing anymore. Our verbal communication clarifies, and it brings us closer together. I am always surprised at how loneliness in families disappears as family members learn communication.

Communication is learned. We've learned the how and the what of communication from the first moment of our lives. By the time we were five years old, we probably have had a billion experiences in sharing communication. We have developed ideas about ourselves, about the world, about other people; we have learned what to expect and how we can communicate to get what was possible.

I see communication as a huge umbrella that covers and affects all that goes on between human beings. Once a human has arrived on this earth, communication is the largest single factor determining what kinds of relationships he makes with others and what happens to him in the world about him. I have found that high self-esteem people communicate directly, openly, and fully. They level with other people, dealing with what is, not what they guess or fear. They send congruent messages. Their voice and words match their facial expressions and their body position. The leveling response occurs when people have relationships that are easy, free, and honest. The leveling response is real. If a leveler says, "I like you," his voice is warm and he looks at you. If his words are, "I am mad as hell at you," his voice is harsh, and his face is tight. The message is simple and straight. I trust a leveler because his messages are truths of the moment. I feel good because I know where I stand with him.

In therapy I use exercises that allow people to feel how they are responding. I developed these ideas from listening to literally thousands of interactions among people. It seems to me that I can let people experience the leveling response by contrasting it to other ways we have of responding. I find that we usually use four other ways besides the leveling. These occur to protect the speaker, rather than primarily to communicate to the listener. In other words, self-esteem is low when these are used.

A person may *placate*, so the other person is happy, does not get mad, and so on.
A person may *blame*, so the other person regards him as strong.
A person may *compute*. He tries to deal with what is by saying that it is harmless, or he tries to protect his self-worth with big words.
A person may *distract*, so the other person does not get any relevant message. The distracter does not respond to the point; he seems dizzily off in different directions. He is purposeless and lonely, but he tries to let nobody know.

For a person to experience the *placater* response, I exaggerate and expand facial and voice messages. I get the placater to feel as he talks to the other person in an ingratiating way, trying to please, apologizing, and never disagreeing no matter what. He is syrupy, martryrish, bootlicking. So that a person can really feel his body during placating, I suggest a stance. I get him to go down physically on one knee, wobble a bit, put out one hand in a begging fashion, be sure to have head up so that neck and shoulders experience placating. Very shortly this placater feels nauseous, if he is listening to himself. He feels strained and headachy. He sounds whiny and squeaky, because he can't get deep breaths. He must get someone to approve of him, and yet this is impossible as long as he says "yes" to everything.

I have the *blamer* stand with one hand on his hip, the other extended with the index finger pointed. Good blamers get bulging neck muscles and flaring nostrils. They also feel their screwed up face and curled lips, as they tell off, call names, and criticize everything under the sun. Blamers disagree, "You never do anything right. What is the matter with you?" Blamers are bosses, but internally they feel unsuccessful, and are confused about their self-esteem.

The *computer* is ultra-reasonable, correct, distant, monotonous and abstract. He says things like, "If one were to observe carefully one might notice the work-worn hands of someone present here." (A leveler could say, "Look at my hands. You can tell I work hard!") The computer uses big words. He is rigid, because he has no feeling from the cranium down. He seems calm, cool, and collected; but deep inside he feels a lack of self-esteem, he feels vulnerable. The sad part about the computer is that many people are taught to be this way as an ideal goal. "Say the right words; show no feeling; don't react." That is advice for a robot, not a human being.

The *distracter*, on the other hand, is most reactive, but his reactions are not relevant to what anyone else is saying or doing. To play the distracter, feel yourself as a kind of lopsided top, constantly spinning, but never knowing where you are going, and not even realizing it when you get there. Distracters have mouth, arms, and legs all moving at once. A few minutes of playing the distracter lets a person experience a terrible loneliness and purposelessness, because the distracter can never be fully present.

Experiencing these four ways of communicating lets people get in touch with their body reactions. Internal feelings experienced in the past come into awareness. These are old ways of communicating, learned perhaps early in childhood. If a person vividly experiences himself in one of these nonfunctional communication patterns, he is better able to reject it. He is acutely conscious of what he needs and wants to reject. He is better able to learn and use the leveling response. As he begins to become more able with the leveling response, his self-esteem goes up and, as his self-esteem goes up, he is still more able to level. He feels confident. And so he is confident as he expresses himself. I hope I am not over-simplifying here. To become a leveler takes, besides someone to show you how, guts, courage, and some new beliefs, too. I don't think you can fake it.

I have found that as a person's self-esteem goes up, and as his self-expression is more able, he begins to realize himself as a whole human being, able to form mutually satisfying relationships that have satisfactory outcomes.

In teaching communication, I am striking out at what I see as the real human evils of this world. For me, the feelings of isolation, helplessness, feeling unloved, low self-esteem or incompetence are the real evils. Certain kinds of communication can change these. I try to make it possible for each person to experience, through the leveling response, his ability to deal directly, spontaneously, congruently and lovingly with others.

The Therapist

I suppose that being genuine is really the most important qualification for a therapist. I find that an effective therapist is genuine to each person in a family. He sees each child as a distinct person, just as he sees each adult as a distinct person. I try to contact each child at eye level to assure that this genuineness, or realness, can flow between us. This means quite a bit of stooping for me, but I think it's important for any child to experience the mutual respect that comes as two people relate closely at eye level. Since first experiences are very important, this eye-to-eye genuineness helps open and develop my relatedness, and so it furthers what I can do as a therapist.

I so see myself as a change agent. I roll up my sleeves and get to work actively helping families change. I try to help them discover the patterns that don't work, and to replace these with patterns that do work. I see a therapist as self-confident, and as curious, too. I go into a family with the attitude of research. I am interested in what actually is going on, not what may seem to be going on, and often not what the family thinks at first they want to be seen as going on. Because of this, I think it is vital that therapists have no blaming attitude about them.

Helping families in trouble emphasizes research and analysis into their particular dynamics for the purpose of help. For example, I may find in a family someone who is hiding behind the boss parental cloak. Sometimes I find a *boss* who is a tyrant. He flaunts his power, knows everything, and parades as a paragon of virtue. He may say, "I am the authority. Family members do as I say." Sometimes I may find a boss who is a martyr. He absolutely wants nothing for himself except to serve the other family members. He will go to astonishing lengths to appear as nothing to be considered. He may say, "Never mind me. Family members, just be happy." Another boss I may find is the Great Stone Face, who lectures incessantly, very impassively, on all the right things. He'll say, "This is the right way."

Now the point of my discoveries, finding such interesting specimens, seems antithetical to most researchers. I am not interested in labeling. My discoveries are for the purpose of knowing what can be done, what can be worked with in a family. All the boss specimens that I have found seem to be suffering from low self-esteem. As a therapist, I'm more confident in beginning to work toward change in the family as I discover each separate individual. Change begins here.

I find that I work best when I have taken time to feel secure about where the separate family members are. Then I sense where I am in relation to this. This helps me to feel comfortable, and I like to feel comfortable in my work. Work goes best when the therapist enjoys what he is doing. In a very real sense, he is having fun. He has a feeling of lightness about what he is accomplishing. In point of fact, I don't think anyone is competent unless, at the same time, he enjoys what he is doing.

I find, too, that as I am genuine and free, expressing my feelings as they occur, family members pick up on this crucial concept: It is safe to express honest feelings. To be even more emphatic about this, I consider 90 percent of a therapist's work is maintaining a counseling climate of safety, the kind of safe atmosphere in which family members feel and act like they feel OK in expressing their feelings. Along with this, I probably should mention again my belief that a therapist must never punish. Punishment does not teach. In the same manner, "Obey me" techniques don't work. Perhaps I mean that therapists teach by deed, not directive. (I recognize that here I am feeling uncomfortable, because I sound too didactic. But this is information, rather than therapy, so I will let it go at that.) This contradiction reminds me that, as therapists, we consciously call the shots as we see them. We deal with the reality, the *what is,* as we perceive it. We have common sense and we use it. We don't accept the surface; we uncover. We trust our bodies too. I have been in families where the air was icy with politeness, or where the air felt stifling to me because of the boredom. I have experienced families in which I felt as dizzy as a spinning top, or families in which there is an air of foreboding, like the lull before a storm, when thunder may crash and lightning may strike at any moment. These troubled atmospheres give me the reactions of back and shoulder aches, head pains, or even a queasy stomach. I find that, by being acutely aware, my body will tell me a lot about a family.

Later when I know the family better, and when they are more healthy, I may share some of my reactions and feelings. One of the all-weather signs of health I find is a sense of humor. When I can look back with a family as they experience the relief of choosing not to go back to dead-end communication, then I feel happy that I am in the presence of health. I understand from my experiences when physical ills must begin. Bodies react humanly to very inhuman atmospheres.

I think the last thing I want to mention about the therapist has a two-fold part. Love and democracy seem related to me, like two parts of one quality. I think good therapists like people with a depth of sincere regard that is love. And they bear this good will to all family members. They democratically accept all family members. A situation that always drives this home to me every time I face it occurs with the child abuser. I see the child abuser as a child grown big, reaching to their own growing up. After my aves of nausea pass, I go to work to help these adults, as ; the children, with their shame, their ignorance and their n. And just as in all good therapy, punishment makes mat- vorse; treatment for these people has to be to help them in ning better persons.

My Goals

lealthy, nurturing families are made up of physically healthy, r ntally alert, feeling, loving, playful, authentic, creative, and p)ductive human beings. These human beings can stand on th eir own two feet; they can love deeply; and they can fight fairly and effectively. They are persons on equally good terms with both their tenderness and their toughness, and they know the difference between the two. These persons compose families in which four things are apparent.

1. Self-worth is high. ✓
2. Communication is direct, clear, specific and honest. ✓
3. Rules are flexible, human and appropriate; they are subject ✓ to change.
4. The linking to society is open and hopeful. ✓

I think that all healthy families have these parts in common. The healthy family is made up of people who value themselves; each esteems himself and the others; and they are conscious of their value as a group. I've found that people of self-esteem know their families are good places to get their needs met. Their homes are nurturing. These people know it is OK to ask for what they need. They can speak openly of their needs, their disappointments, their achievements, their dreams. Because needs change, really from minute to minute, these people chose rules for their families that accommodate them, that are suitable to them. They find themselves as the value, and so do not arbitrarily follow rules. These people are energetic questioners, too. They are constantly asking: Does it fit? Does this rule, or way of relating in our family, further growth? Does our family encourage our getting our needs met both here, and in the world? In other words, is our linking to society open and hopeful, so that we may expect to have a good time in the world?

Family rules are vital, dynamic, influential forces. These rules are the force that either slows you down or gets you on your way. The importance of these rules just cannot be emphasized too much. In fact, I would say that helping individuals and families to discover the rules by which they live is my goal—and I think it's surprising to families to discover their rules. Many families are not even aware of their rule system.

Rules have to do with *should*. Rules also abbreviate what is possible. Rather than beginning anew each time the possibility for a decision or a choice or an action comes up, families depend upon their shoulds. Family members don't have to make a new decision each time on what money is to be used for, who does chores, or what to do about infractions.

A good way that I have for discovering the rules of a family is to have all family members present, and to have them sit down and write their rules. Two hours is about enough time. The family may appoint a secretary if they chose. Now is not the time for argument, nor discussion. Have all the family members add what they think their rules are. Maybe this family has a 10-year old boy who thinks the rule is that he only has to wash the dishes when his 11-year old sister is justifiably occupied somewhere else. He figures he is a kind of back-up dishwasher. His sister thinks the rule is that her brother washes the dishes when his father tells him to. It's easy to see misunderstanding resulting here. I listen to irate parents tell me, "He knows what the rules are!" But I frequently find that's not the case.

Actually seeing their rules written out helps a family to see whether their rules are fair and appropriate. They can see if their rights are up-to-date. A nurturing family keeps up-to-date rules; and they are adaptable. Our legal system provides for appeals; I think good family rule systems do, too.

After acknowledging what their rules are, a family can confront the question of who makes the rules. Is it the person who is the oldest, the nicest, the most handicapped, the most powerful? Are rules from books, from TV shows, from neighbors or from the families where the parents grew up?

A good family rule system allows freedom to comment on what is, not on what should be. I deal with four aspects of this freedom of comment.

First, I try to get the answer to: What can you say about what you're seeing and hearing? Expressing fear, helplessness, anger, need for comfort, loneliness, tenderness or aggression forms some of the blocks. Then, I want to know: To whom can you say it? I may find some disjunction - like the child who hears a parent swearing, and there is a family rule against swearing. The child may not remind the parent, yet the parent must remind the child if it were the other way around.

After this, I need to know: How do you go about it if you disagree or disapprove of someone or something? If your 69-year old grandmother always loses the phone book, can you say so?

My fourth question is: How do you question when you don't understand? Of course, many families don't question at all when they don't understand, but families can learn that they can get clarification. They can get understanding, and they can be understood.

All kinds of seeing and hearing go on in families. My goal is to get family members to use all their seeing and hearing for closeness, for trust, for support and for joy. Even though secrets having to do with deformity, jail, illegitimacy, and so on may exist, talking around a subject, or hiding the secret, does not remove it. Only talking about good, right, appropriate subjects leaves out large parts of reality. These shutting-off attitudes breed low self-esteem, because any family member who is asked in any way to deny his perceptions will be hurt.

The area probably most often placed out-of-touch, or denied, is that of sex. Some families deny that sexual beings, males and females, compose their family. One's sexuality has a vast influence on one's separate individuality. This is important because uniqueness is the key word to self-worth. The family is the place to learn that it is good to be a female, or that it is good to be a male. I have had contact with family rules as stringent as: Don't enjoy sex—yours or anyone else's—in any form.

Some families see genitals as necessary nasty objects. Because so much pain comes from repression and inhuman attitudes about sex, I try to get attitudes changed to pride, openness, acceptance, enjoyment and appreciation. I can say that, without exception, any person I have seen with problems in sexual gratification in marriage, or who was promiscuous, or who was arrested for any sexual crime grew up with some taboos against sex. I'll go further. Anyone whom I have seen with any kind of coping problem or emotional illness also grew up with taboos about sex.

So I believe that anything that is can be talked about and understood in human terms. My goal is to get family members to realize that expressing themselves honestly gets them in deepest touch with themselves, and with each other, and this means they stand a much better chance of creating satisfying relationships with the outside world.

Now to touch briefly on something I mentioned when I began to talk of goals. With people of self-worth, full sharing respects dreams. I see dreams as the force or impetus of life. Dreams give life something to flow toward. And it seems to me that when a person's dreams—his wants, his desires—become confidence, he is doing and enjoying doing. He confidently acts his dreams. Family sharing can help this come about.

Illustrative Protocol

The protocol below is from a Symposium on Family Counseling and Therapy that I participated in. When we began, we worked on a stage. It seemed we had some uncomfortable family members, so I tried to get each member of the family seated in a comfortable way with his feet upon something secure. As we began to talk, I discovered that Elaine was 4, Jimmy was 6, Jane was 10, and Mary was 11. The parents, John and Alice, were 42 and 34 at that time. I'd been around for 54 years, so I mentioned that we had a conglomerate of experiences to draw from. We talked of expectations, and then something of family home activity. The family had volunteered, from John's point of view, to learn something about their own family dynamics. The positions referred to as the protocol begins are those that occurred when I grouped the family members close to the persons within the family that each was close to. The arrangement of the two oldest on either side of John, and the two youngest on either side of Alice seemed comfortable to the family. I had begun by trying to get at how they, as a family, lived. We have been working about fifteen minutes; now we are learning about some behavior rules.

John: Alice is not nearly as strict with them as I am. I think she would agree with that, and yet her control with them is much better than mine.

Jane: He blows his top.

Satir: He blows his top. All right, all right. But I did feel something change. Did you see something change when you changed your positions? Alice, what kind of explanations would you give for that?

Alice: I guess these two *(Mary and Jane)* feel as if they don't have to stay within certain bounds when they're with me as they do when they're with him. That's the only explanation that I have. I'm not so good at blowing my top, I guess.

Satir: Do you want to get better?

Alice: I guess so. I mean, I don't know if that would be the solution. I would like to be firmer with them, but I don't want to go into the anger and so forth that is involved with it. We're just so different. I mean, he is a very emotional person and he reacts to every little thing. He just flares up and I don't.

Satir: You know, just let me tell you something that I was feeling. It may or may not be right that sometimes you ask yourself if you ought to be different from what you are when you don't really believe it. I don't think you really believe you'd like to blow your top, would you?

Alice: Not blow my top. I would like to be able to be more positive.

Satir: Could you give me an example of what you mean by that?

Alice: I would like to be able to say, "No, you are not going to do this," and then make it stick - to be convincing with the children.

Satir: John, what are your feelings as you hear Alice talk at this moment?

John: She and I think differently about this. I'm firmly convinced... Let me use an analogy. I would not teach without a paddle. I only had to use it three times in 16 years, but it was there. I feel that a recourse to this is necessary. I believe that if you are going to tell somebody something you'd better not tell them anything that you don't enforce, because pretty soon they begin to lose the credibility of it. I feel like that many times she tells them to do things and she doesn't mean to enforce it or, at least, she does not enforce it the way I do.

Satir: Alice do you get that picture? At least that is how John sees you.

Alice: Well, so many times it's just easier to do it myself.

Satir: Well, how do you feel about his idea?

Alice: I think many times he is too harsh.

Satir: And what kinds of problems does that make for you?

Alice: Ground-out teeth.

Satir: Ground-out teeth. Would you be willing to try something?

Alice: I guess.

Satir: Would you, John?

John: Let me make one comment. One of the things that I notice, and I think its important, is that when they (*Jane and Jimmy and Mary and Elaine*) do divide it's a result of these two (*Jane and Mary*) competing. When you talk about tension, this is a more tension-free arrangement, because the competition in the other arrangement does cause tension. But, now let's get on to what you were saying.

Satir: Okay, Elaine, what I'm going to ask you to do is just to let your chair move back a little bit and yours too, Jane. I'd like you to be in a theater somewhere, just watching. If you can stay where you are, I'll put you face-to-face. Now we'll just try this out for size, okay? Alice, I wonder if you could say to John: "I think you're too harsh."

Alice: I think you're too harsh.

Satir: Now, John, would you respond to her?

John: I do my best.

Satir: Alice, how did you feel about what he told you?

Alice: Well, he does do his best. I think he needs to relax more, though.

Satir: He didn't answer you regarding your disagreeing with his harshness though, did he? How did you feel about his not answering that?

Alice: It's a typical answer.

Satir: All right. Let's try it again and you say to him again that you feel he is too harsh.

Alice: I think you're too harsh.

John: I think that I need recourse to violence to make them behave, and I do what I think is right.

Satir: All right, now would you try again. When you *(Alice)* tell him that you think he is too harsh, will you *(John)* say to her that you believe that she's wrong.

Alice: I think you are too harsh.

John: I think you're wrong.

Satir: Alice, how do you want to respond to that?

Alice: I think I'm right.

John: I see a fight starting!

Satir: Now, John, you're laughing about it, but could you tell me now how that makes you feel when this comes up?

John: This doesn't come up.

Satir: I noticed that. I know why. I think it needs to, though. All right, could you respond, John? Alice said that she thinks she's right.

John: I think you're wrong.

Alice: This could go on indefinitely.

Satir: Yeah, and this is one of the things out of which there would be no escape, once this happened. Right? Oh, the kids can do it instead. All right, would you move a little closer? Alice, would you just look at him and tell him something that you know that you and he absolutely agree on.

Alice: We need to get off and have some time, just to ourselves.

John: Amen.

Satir: Does that mean you agree?

John: Yes ma'am.

Satir: All right, you tell her that you agree with her.

John: I just did.

Satir: No, now you sounded like a preacher.

John: *(to Alice)* I thoroughly agree, wholeheartedly.

Satir: Now, Alice, what does that make you want to do?

Alice: Well, I wish we could make some plans to get away.

Satir: Would you tell him something that you want to do with him.

Alice: Well, this really is what we had been planning - to take a little vacation.

Satir: Is it set up?

Alice: Yes, tentatively.

Satir: All right, now what could stop it?

Alice: Child-care problems.

Satir: Okay, now would you discuss your child-care problems?

Alice: We live too far away from either set of grandparents, so we'll have to try and make arrangements to have a friend come in and stay at the house with the children or "farm them out" either in small groups or separately among our friends. We'll be gone about three days.

Satir: How soon is this going to be?

Alice: April.

Satir: April. All right, now you named several possibilities, different children going to different places, and so forth. Would you discuss together, at this point in time, given the information that you have, what you think would be a likely plan.

Alice: Well I've thought of several things.

Alice and John continue to agree, working out plans. Now I have gotten back to one place they need help. We're working on their disagreeing with each other, rather than their disagreeing through the children.

Satir: I see, so there is something that scares you about the whole business of the disagreement.

John: Very much!

Satir: What about you, Alice? What objections do you have to disagreeing with John?

Alice: Well, it's unpleasant, for one thing.

Satir: Could you go further with that, dear?

Alice: Whatever problems we have, I feel that we could find a better solution than the constant disagreeing and bickering.

Satir: Now let's do something, because one of the problems that I see here is that there is something pretty horrible about the whole business of disagreeing in the family. You haven't found yet a growth way to use the disagreement. So let's play around with something. Maybe by the time we leave we'll be able to know something different about this disagreement.

John: Let me make one comment to Alice that this is by no means an uncommon thing. I just want to tell her that this happens in every family.

Satir: I hear you trying to give Alice some reassurance, John, that she's not so different from other people and neither are you.

John: Essentially, yes.

Satir: John, could you find some ways to talk more simply to Alice?

John: It's difficult for me to talk simply.

Satir: Yeah, every once in a while I have a feeling that I want to get out the dictionary. But anyway, you said that you started out by placating during disagreements.

John: Now this was a number of years ago.

Satir: Long ago?

John: Now she is reasonable.

Satir: Well, would you take the placating stance. Alice, do you remember when he was saying, "Yes dear," to you, a long time ago?

Alice: No.

Satir: Well, John, this is your recall of this. Which one of these in front of you would you be saying "yes" to.

John: Her *(Alice)*.

Satir: Alice. Well, Alice, now you may not have known this, but apparently this was true. Now, John, how did you see Alice reacting when you did this? Blaming, all right. Alice, this may not be your picture, but it is his picture of you. John, what does it feel like for you down there in a placating position?

John: Door mat.

Satir: So you raged inside then. Alice, if you never knew that this was going on, then this could be a whole piece of John that you didn't know about. Now, John, breathe a little, because otherwise you'll get a backache. When you see that stance, Alice, what do you find yourself doing? Is it that way or is it "To hell with you brother" kind of thing? Okay, so you do go "To hell with you brother," and you do what I say. . .with the finger pointed this way. Is that something you've seen, John?

John: Not that reasonable stance.

Satir: Well, wait a minute, though; this time you talk about what you feel, so you apparently haven't seen this.

John: No, I haven't.

Satir: You see it is hard because Alice is looking over there. Alice, would you notice where your finger is going?

Alice: I can't see.

Satir: No you can't see, but you can feel it from behind. You really want to say to him, "Get off my back" Okay, so he did. Now, John, when you said that you finally stopped; it is very understandable why you stopped and assumed the "reasonable guy" stance. What does that make you want to do, Alice?

Alice: I would like to communicate, to tell him not to be so reasonable.

Satir: Okay, so what do you want?

John: She hasn't decided yet.

Alice: You talk for me.

Satir: What is it for you? All right, you are at this point now. Alice what do you see yourself doing?

Alice: Not placating, but something similar to that. Pleading. It is not quite as much as that.

Satir: All right then kind of like this! You look straight at him. You kind of bend your knees a little and appear to be saying "Please look at me, please." All right, children I would like to ask you if you ever have seen these position between your mother and dad when he stands like a solid rock of Gibraltar?

Jane: Sometimes.

Satir: What do you find yourself doing when that happens? What do you find happening? What do you feel like you're doing? Do you kind of stand stiff, too? What's your picture?

Jane: *(Jane pushes her father)*

Satir: Do you really want to wipe it all out? Push him away. All right, just stand kind of like you want to push him away. Now John, you're kind of pleading down here. Where do you think you are? All right, you hold that position for a minute. Elaine, where do you think you are, dear? You're up there too. You want to say you are with your father, huh? Okay and you've already felt that the two of you are together. Is this something in your family that you've noticed? Jane really tries to get you two to stop.

Jane: I don't like you *(father)* but.

Satir: All right, Jane is in-between.

John: Jane tries to control in our situation.

Satir: Alice, have you noticed this?

Alice: Yes.

Satir: All right, have you seen this in relation to Mary?

Alice: Yes, but not that stance.

Satir: Okay, we're exaggerating this stance, but have you seen this, John?

John: Not clearly.

Satir: Not clearly. Is it beginning to come through now?

Mary: I tell dad what to do. I tell him to be nicer to mommy and I tell her to be nicer to him.

Satir: Well, wait a minute now. There are a lot of pieces here. All right, you can put your arm down further. What I heard you say is that you tick your dad off and say, "Now, look, you be nicer to mother." Is that it?

Mary: I tell him what to do to her. I tell him what she'd like...

Satir: All right, you do that right now. Will you tell your father out loud so we can all hear?

Mary: Daddy, when you talk to mommy, she can't take all that yelling. Next time you feel like yelling, just ask yourself, "Would mommy like the way I say it or would she dislike it?" Just try not to yell.

Satir: Alice, is this something you yourself have been experiencing from Mary?

Alice: Not in those words.

Satir: *(to Mary)* You want to tell your dad, "Please be nicer to mommy." All right now. Mary, go over to your mother and tell her what you want to tell her.

Mary: You shouldn't yell.

Alice: I don't yell that much.

Satir: Now Mary, you are saying to your mother, "You be nicer to daddy. He can't help it."

Mary: He can't help it that he yells so much.

Satir: Alice, have you noticed this happening?

Alice: Yes, in a very...

Satir: This is only one piece of it. What we're getting at is that when this family reaches a rupture, which is when the two of you have problems where you are objecting and disagreeing, then here is one way that this family operates. Mary is trying to give her father some advice about how to treat his wife, and Mary is trying to give her mother some advice about how to understand her husband. That's what I hear.

As we continued the interview, their network of rules continued to come out. We worked on clear communication, and fair disagreements that do not contradict the love family members have for each other. We worked on the family problem of rules coming from supposed to. Because this interview uncovered so much, follow-up work was done with the family, so they could better resolve their concerns.

Summary

Family therapy is, of course, for families; although I have noticed that three or more people related in any way that are joined by a common task will develop into a family system. So this type of therapy is theoretically suitable for many small groups. I think that, when we are in groups, we shape ourselves into families because for so long the family has been the basic social unit. It almost goes without saying that I think the family still is the basic social unit, and that it will remain so. I see the family as the place where a person can sit down and be known. The family is a small enough group for this. Most families do not exceed the recognized full-group number of 15. In the family group, each person is appreciated for his unique value. Each person has a unique place. These places all are at different growth levels. These places balance and accommodate each other.

To give a family group an experience of how they accommodate each other and balance each other, I sometimes provide objects— any objects that are very different from one another. The family is to work out a mobile, to create their mobile by balancing the different objects. There should be as many objects as there are people in the family. Some families will settle for the first balance they achieve; I try to encourage at least three solutions, pointing out the interest and variety. One of the points in the exercise is to see that just as moving one part of the mobile to another place affects all other places, family members do not rearrange themselves without affecting the whole group. Families who become conscious, thoughtful of others, will have members who consider before changing the family pattern.

I think it's very important to realize that so much family change is what I call *normal crisis.* These are the natural stresses that are predictable for most people. The crises contain temporary anxiety, require an adjustment period, and require a new integration. After a male and a female decide to begin a family, their first child is their first crisis. There is the conception, pregnancy, and birth. Being the first child is part of the crisis, because he is the guinea pig. I do not see how it can be otherwise.

A second normal crisis occurs when this child starts to use intelligible speech. This second crisis requires a big adjustment. The third crisis occurs when the child goes to school. The fourth crisis is big. This is when the child enters adolescence. The fifth crisis is when the child has grown to adulthood, and he leaves home. There are heavy loss feelings here. The sixth comes when the young adult marries, expanding the family by adding in-laws. The seventh is the advent of menopause in the woman. The eighth is the climacteric for the man. This crisis is unpredictable, and seems to spring more from the male's idea that he is losing his potency than with anything physical. The ninth comes with grand-parenting, which is chock full of privileges and traps. Finally, the tenth comes when death comes to one of the spouses and then to the other.

The changes are normal and rapid. More change goes on in families at a quicker rate than in any other social group that I can think of. Three or four crises may cluster at once, and can indeed make life "worriable."

Frequently, this is when families come for help. If a family has not expected change-emerging differences, if they have cultivated a static condition and homogeneity, they run the risk of falling flat on their faces, and they do need help to get back up. People get born, grow big, work, marry, become parents, grow old and die. In my therapy I try to create awareness and increase communication skills to help families adjust and grow with the squeezes and stresses of life.

Research

I am now using a structured interview in six major ways:

1. It provides a method of structuring family behavior and of developing ways of classifying family behavior. Hopefully, our raw data on family behavior will lead to the formulation of appropriate concepts in which we can describe families. Clearly, one of the difficulties in analyzing an individual's behavior, using my system and communication approach, is that we do not have clear and universal terms in which to describe family systems and family rules.

2. The interview can be used to compare different families task-by-task, and so on.

3. Families may be compared with themselves, at the beginning and end of treatment.
4. The interview information may be compared with the information and insight that therapy brings out.
5. The interview may be used diagnostically, indicating guidelines for therapy.
6. The interview is part of the therapy. Responding clearly to the interview is a therapeutic experience for a family if it breaks some of their dysfunctional rules—their growth inhibiting, distorting or assaulting rules. Observing that a catastrophe does not follow direct, level responses forms an important experience for some family members.

Dr. Jules Riskin is working on a set of scales to describe and classify interaction. These scales attempt to show such things as clarity versus congruency, or does what is said match how it is said. The scales will deal with concepts like commitment versus avoiding commitment, agreeing or disagreeing, and increased or decreased intensity. So far, his results suggest meaningful and significant variables of interaction.

Another investigator, Jay Haley, is trying to develop a more mechanical method for differentiating families and measuring interaction. He uses a four-minute sequence of a three-person interchange (father, mother, child) and records the speaking order. Who speaks after whom is significantly different, in that the order is more rigid in disturbed families. His research has the implication that the family does show patterns, an implication that supports my idea that the family is a system.

The general goal of research is learning to describe, identify, and then use the system for the growth of all family members. The results, with both normal and pathogenic families, suggest that we are beginning.

References

Jackson, D., and Satir, V. (1961). A method of analysis of a family interview. *Archives of General Psychiatry.* 5 (4), 321 – 339. Chicago: American Medical Association.

Jackson, D., and Satir, V. (1962). A review of psychiatric developments in family diagnosis and family therapy. *Exploring the Base for Family Therapy.* New York: Family Service Association.

Satir, V. (1963). *Conjoint family therapy.* Palo Alto, CA: Science and Behavior Books.

Satir, V. (1965). The Family as a Treatment Unit. *Confina Psychiatrica.* Basel S. Karger. New York: Basel S. Karger. Vol. 8, pp. 37-42.

Satir, V. (1970). I am me. *Etcetera: A Review of General Semantics.* 11 (4), 463-464.

Satir, V. (1971). Conjoint family therapy: Demonstration with a Family. [Videotape] *Proceedings of a Symposium on Training Groups.* The University of Georgia: College of Education.

Satir, V. Demonstration With Nine Volunteers. (1971). [Audiotape] *Proceedings of a symposium on training groups.* The University of Georgia: College of Education.

Satir, V. (1971). Symptomatology: A family production. *Theory and Practice of Family Psychiatry.* John G. Howells. New York: Brunner/Mazel.

Satir, V. (1972). *Peoplemaking.* Palo Alto, CA: Science and Behavior Books.

Warshofsky, Fred. (1971). An Interview with Virginia Satir. *Family Circle*, November, 42-43.

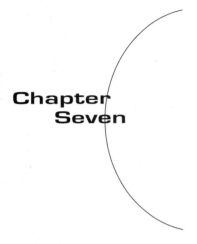

Chapter Seven

A Partial Portrait of a Family Therapist in Process

Introduction by Colleen Murphy

In "Partial Portrait...", Virginia Satir shares not only the internal and external contexts of her professional growth but also her understanding of a health-oriented, positive psychology perspective, the survival stances, the mandala, family and social systems, the survival purpose of symptoms, the Life Energy of the Self, and the necessity of the congruence of the therapist. These concepts are all discussed in this article, as are the processes through which they came to be understood. The concepts themselves were unique contributions at the time that Satir was practicing as a Family Therapist but perhaps none was more pivotal and more predictive of what was to come in our profession than her focus on the personhood of the therapist.

If a profession can be said to have elders, ancestors who provide a guiding light from the past as we move inexorably into the future, then Satir begins her "Partial Portrait" by acknowledging our elders. She describes her own context of evolution as a therapist in terms of her esteemed colleagues, including Bateson, Bowen, Ackerman, Riskin, Erickson, Minuchin and others, who are some of our recognized forefathers today.

Throughout, Satir's language reflects the wholeness and evolution of her beliefs as she moved beyond the psychopathology mores of the day to a core belief in health. She "clung to a bone-deep conviction ... family members could be in real contact with one an-

other" Satir places her current (1982) knowing in its time and casts an encouraging light forward for the continued evolution of our profession of family therapy and of ourselves as family therapists.

Quoting what Satir says in this chapter: "Some of the past discoveries were buds that had to be developed. And some were basic new discoveries. It will go on that way. It has been that way for me."

Antithetical to the thinking of the time, Satir held that new and seemingly contradictory ideas are enriching. She suggests that through the various schools of family therapy we work together as opposed to attempting to define the one most "right" way.

In "Partial Portrait," Satir truly demonstrates what a visionary she has been in the practice of Family Therapy. What we now take almost for granted—such as the role of the therapist and his/ her beliefs in the therapeutic process, positive psychology vs. psychopathology, the holistic approach to mental and emotional health, how much we still have to learn about the mystery of being human—Satir recognized and articulated decades ago.

In closing, Satir locates her emphasis on us, family therapists, on our integrity, our openness to new information, our willingness to go beyond the boundaries of what has been learned thus far. She suggests not that we follow in her footsteps or the footsteps of our other ancestors, but rather that we follow their spirit and step forward on our own paths, with competence, confidence and congruence.

■ ■ ■

I am one of the first in a small group of homemade, untrained family therapists who made their appearance in the 1950's. All of the early pioneers (including myself) in what led to what we are now calling family therapy felt challenged by and/or cared about the "hopeless" schizophrenic population. What we learned was expanded and modified into what we are all doing today. I want to speak briefly about eight of these people. I am aware there are others. I am selecting those who were best known to me.

Kalman Gyarfas, M.D., a Hungarian-born psychiatrist and a beautiful caring man, was then Superintendent of the Chicago State Hospital. He felt some of the answer to schizophrenia lay in the family. When the program was first being developed for the

Illinois State Psychiatric Institute in Chicago in March 1955, where Dr. Gyarfas was also in charge, he asked me to teach the residents what I knew about family dynamics, my forerunner to family therapy. By that time I had been seeing families for nearly four years. As an influence in the development of family therapy, Dr. Gyarfas is hardly known outside of Chicago. He put his efforts into helping the psychiatric residents see the patient within the family context.

In 1956, I sought contact with Murray Bowen, M.D. who, along with Warren Brody, M.D. and Bob Dysinger, M.D., was researching families with schizophrenic members who were hospitalized at the National Institute of Mental Health. He graciously invited me to visit him. Dr. Bowen came out of his research with a theory of family ego mass and developed a way of changing families through dealing with the one he perceived as the "governor" of the system. He has expanded that to look at intergenerational systems.

Nathan Ackerman, whom I did not meet until 1962, had the kernels of how a symptomatic family member connects with other family members. He wrote about this in 1934 and then apparently left that orientation until the middle fifties when he started clinical work with whole families.

I became acquainted with Don Jackson through his article called "Toward a Theory of Schizophrenia" in the fall of 1956 (Bateson et al., 1956). I remember that when I read that article I nearly fell off my chair with excitement. He was describing phenomena that I was seeing. I recognized then how isolated and out of the main stream I had been feeling. Here was a fellow traveler. (To many of the professional community in Chicago, where I was living and working at that time, I appeared as a freak. Probably because I was a nice freak, I was still accepted.) I came to know later that Dr. Jackson was working with Gregory Bateson, Jay Haley, and others who were later associated with the Mental Research Institute (MRI) in Palo Alto, California. Dr. Jackson's article made such an impression on me that, when I came to California in early 1959, I called him. He invited me to present for his group In Palo Alto. It was that day that he asked me to join him and Dr. Jules Riskin to form MRI. The three of us opened MRI on March 19, 1959. We focused on communication, looking at the double-bind theory, as well as other communication concepts.

Jay Haley exclusively emphasized what went on between people. He was actually looking at the destructive uses of power, and attempted to make individuals' use of themselves conscious so that people could employ more positive power tactics to get what they needed and wanted. He was much influenced by Dr. Milton Erickson and the whole one-upmanship theory.

Salvador Minuchin, as a young psychiatrist, worked with Dr. Ed Auerswald at the Wiltwyck School for Boys. This school was for the delinquent sons of largely one-parent black families. On the surface, one might have looked at these people as hopeless. Dr. Minuchin saw the resources within these families and mobilized them so that the families could come to better places. He, in a sense, was the first one who demonstrated that the so-called hopeless ones in this population could be substantially helped. Since there was such a need for members of these families to structure their lives, Dr. Minuchin emphasized structure and working out the power lines. Many of the parents in these families had no notion of how they could view and use themselves differently. He gave them hope and tools.

I first met Dr. Minuchin in the middle sixties when he invited me to come to Wiltwyck School to share whatever I had with him. Our paths have joined, separated, and rejoined at different points, depending on our levels of accord or disagreement. I have a profound respect for this man who saw hope where there seemed to be none, and proceeded to give it a reality.

Carl Wittaker, M.D., one of the early members of the Peachtree Group in Atlanta, Georgia, is also a deeply respectful, loving man who can enter into crazy-making systems and change those systems without any of the craziness rubbing off on him.

Gregory Bateson probably contributed more to me about the understanding of human communication than any one else. He, too, was a loving, caring man who was also a brilliant researcher and theorist. I had the good fortune to have known and worked with him.

Whatever I have said about the previously mentioned people is all too brief and represents my own biases, gratitude, and affection.

I was trained as a social worker. My formal training regarding the nature of human beings was exclusively in individual psychoanalytic theory. When I first stumbled on seeing families, I had a thriving private clinical practice. I had had nine years of clinical practice in agencies and six years of elementary and secondary school teaching experience. The therapeutic climate then was rigid and controlled by the medical profession. As a privately practicing nonmedical clinician, I often got the clients no one else wanted or who already had been seen unsuccessfully by a succession of other therapists. That meant I had very difficult and high-risk people to deal with. Being nonmedical, and thus being ineligible for liability insurance, I could not risk casualties. Since private practice was my livelihood, I needed to be successful. Being interested in people, I wanted to see them get well. I had to be a responsible, accountable, competent risk-taking therapist.

I saw my first family in 1951. I was referred a 26-year old woman who had been diagnosed as an "ambulatory schizophrenic." She had seen many therapists with little success.

I was working, literally by the seat of my pants, experimenting with ways to reach her. I put as much of my own learning as I could on the shelf about what schizophrenia was and how treatment was supposed to be. I put myself in an observing position and, basically, let my intuition guide me, tempered of course by my logic. There was nothing written or talked about then in relation to working with families. I had to make up my own guidelines.

After about six months of treatment, when the young woman had improved immeasurably, her mother telephoned me, threatening me with a lawsuit for alienation of affections. For some reason, that day I heard two messages in the mother's voice: a verbal threat and a non-verbal plea. I chose to respond to her plea and to ignore her threat. I invited her to come in. This was an outrageous thing for me to do back then. Yet, she accepted my invitation.

The first time that both the mother and the daughter were together in my office, I noticed something exceedingly unusual. Within minutes after the mother's appearance, my patient was behaving just as she had when I first began seeing her. I was stupefied. I simply couldn't believe what I saw. Nothing in my training had prepared me for this. The only thing I knew to do was to keep my mouth shut and observe.

I noticed an affective clueing operation going on through voice tone, looks, and gestures that was completely inconsistent with the verbal messages. This was the beginning of my awareness of, and understanding of, communication, and became a tap root in my theory and practice. I was seeing the double-level and double-bind messages that were later described so well by Don Jackson, Gregory Bateson, and the MRI group.

When I recovered from my initial shock, I worked in some way with the mother and the daughter until they came to a new balance between them. At some point, it occurred to me that the young woman might have a father, and the mother a husband. Upon inquiry, I found this to be true. In those days, fathers were not really seen as a part of the emotional life of the family, so therapists did not usually think about them. Mothers, on the other hand, were considered to be of primary influence—mostly bad—and so even though they were not seen during the treatment of a child, they were counted.

I asked the mother and the daughter if the father might join us. They accepted my invitation, which they were "not supposed" to do. According to the thinking of the times, they were supposed to have vigorously resisted the idea. The father did come in, and then I had another jolting shock. Both the mother and the daughter were back to their original places.

Again I observed. And I saw the rudiments of coalitions within the primary triad (father, mother, child). This observation later became the first link to my seeing the family as a system. It also led me to look at the power plays in the triad. I worked with these three until a new balance among them was made.

Then the older "perfect son" made his appearance. When he came in, the same imbalance again occurred. I worked with that until a new balance was reached. Shortly after that, treatment was finished. My follow-up information was that the new balance was holding and things were going well.

I cannot tell you now exactly what I did to change that situation, except that I clung to a bone-deep conviction that all these family members could be in real contact with one another and speak congruently with each other. Being convinced that was possible, it was achieved. Then I had to figure out what I did. I had been groping in the dark. What I do remember clearly is that the dynamics I saw were brand new to me. I never dreamed those kinds of goings-on existed. What I learned from that family I used with other families as I went along.

That early period was an exciting one for those of us beginning to look at families, for we were breaking new ground. It was scary venturing beyond the pale because we were theoreticall— and sometimes literally—putting our professional reputations on the line. Since I was nonmedical, I did not get much criticism or have that much to lose.

At the outset, most of us were working in isolation and were not in touch with what others were doing. Since all of us were dealing with schizophrenia, which was considered more or less untreatable anyway, we were initially on the fringe of the psychiatric community.

In the current psychotherapeutic context of 1982, when family therapy is a respected and acceptable mode of therapy, it would be hard for someone who had not lived through that early period to imagine what it was like then.

There are now schools of family therapy, the followers of which argue both subtly and explicitly about who has the right approach. For myself, I feel we would do better to be exchanging our work and building together, for I feel that working with the family is the beginning to fathoming the mysteries of the world.

I feel that what I have learned about families had its beginnings in working with the so called "helpless" schizophrenic people. That first family I have described was very significant to me, and I soon found other families coming out of the rafters. There were so many of them who asked for my help. By 1955, when I started teaching at the Illinois State Psychiatric Institute, I had seen nearly 300 families.

I repeatedly saw the same phenomena I described in that first family in these later families. Later still, when I worked with families with delinquent members, and later yet when I worked with families who had psychosomatic or physically ill members, I saw other variations of the same theme.

By that time, I had freed myself to look at the ways I could help people to get in touch with themselves, and I allowed myself to experiment with anything that I thought could help. I drew on my experience in education, drama, art, general semantics, plant life, and philosophy, as well as what I knew about individual development.

One particular way I found useful was to make body pictures of what was going on in a family. That meant putting the family member's bodies in postures that represented feelings. It meant showing relationships with gestures. When I learned enough about the kind of exaggerated communication that goes with disharmony and dysfunction, I worked out a series of physical postures of what I saw as the basic survival needs of persons coming from a place of low self-esteem. It turned out that those postures were universal. I called the postures stances, and named them placating, blaming, and irrelevant. Later I added the super-reasonable stance.

I do not see my task here as that of detailing all the things I learned that I use today. I want only to say that once I went beyond the boundaries of what I learned about psychopathology and was able to look, instead, at health, I was indeed on a different track.

Over the past 30 years, I have been privileged to work with thousands of families in all economic, social, political, racial and nationality groups from all over the world. I have also taught hundreds of therapists. And, in the course of all that experience, I have made a 180 degree turn in my thinking about people, in and out of families, and in my approach to treatment.

At this time, I see that my therapeutic task lies in reshaping and transforming into useful purposes the energy bottled up in a person's or a family's demonstrated pathology. This is in contrast to my earlier belief that my task was limited to exterminating the pathology. I refer to my present approach as a health-oriented approach, although it is really more than that. I call it the Human Validation Process Model. In this article, I will be using the term *pathology-oriented approach* to mean symptom extermination. *Health oriented approach* will mean the transforming of energy that I referred to above.

To further illustrate the point, I give the following analogy: Let us imagine a wheel with a hub at its center and spokes reaching out to a rim. The spokes represent the various parts of a person. The rim represents the boundaries of a person. I'll talk more about the hub below.

In a pathology oriented approach, one starts with emphasis on the pathology/symptom, the hub, making it the center of one's attention. Thus, one selects out in an individual only that which is destructive and symptom related.

In a health oriented approach, I see the hub as the potential health of the individual present but untapped, covered over, and therefore out of reach to that person. In this frame of thinking, the symptom is an attempt to express that health, even though the individual, by his beliefs and rules, blocks the manifestation of that health.

At this point, I see eight different levels comprising health. They loosely correspond to the spokes of the wheel. Listed, they are:

1. Physical; the body.
2. Intellectual; the left brain, thoughts, facts.
3. Emotional; the right brain, feelings, intuition

4. Sensual; the ears sound, the eyes sight, the nose smell, the mouth taste, and the skin tactile sensation touch movement.
5. Interactional; the I - Thou, communication between oneself and others, and communication between the self and the self.
6. Nutritional; the solids and fluids ingested.
7. Contextual; colors, sound, light, air, temperature, forms, movement, space and time.
8. Spiritual; one's relationship to the meaning of life, the soul, spirit, life force.

Starting with the spiritual part and going toward the physical part, I will elaborate on these levels.

Our Spiritual Dimension

No human being has been able yet to create life. Parents do not create life. They only activate the creation of life through joining a sperm and an egg, the carriers of life. This being true, we all have to face the fact that there is a life force from which all living things come, and that no human being had an active part in inventing. What one calls that force is irrelevant. It is present and the base of our existence. When there is a disturbance, a void, or a conflict in an individual's spiritual dimension, difficulties ensue.

Our Contextual Dimension

Because each individual is always in a context, she or he is always being affected by the light, color, sound, movement, temperature, form, space and time present in that context. When it is too cold, too hot, too drab, too fast, too crowded, too isolated, too late or too early, too quiet, too noisy, too polluted etc., then the individual is subtly affected. For example, we hear that today people have more hearing impairment than before. We have more noise to contend with. We also know that some colors promote harmony; others cause disharmony. The angles and curves of buildings affect us, etc.

Our Nutritional Dimension

It seems we have always known that what we take into our bodies as food and liquids affects our bodies. Doctors have always prescribed special diets for sick people. The idea has been that special foods or liquids can help a sick body get well. But now we are learning that good nutrition can contribute to health of not just the body, but also the mind, the emotions and the other levels. We see that normally healthy people can get healthier by paying attention to their nutrition. Good nutrition contributes to well being. Poor nutrition contributes to poor being, even when the person is actually sick.

Our Interactional Dimension

Every human being came from two other people. We were born essentially into a group. This probably accounts for what appears to be an inborn need to be in touch with other human beings. Because we were born little, we were in a life and death relationship with our parents, the big ones. As infants we had no ability to survive on our own, and we had to put our survival in the hands of other persons. We had, even as infants, needs greater than just physical care. We all had and have needs to be cared for, loved and respected by others. This puts all of us in a vulnerable position with others, and puts a tremendous burden on our links with other people.

Our ongoing work in the world requires that we work with other people in capacities of trust and competence. When that doesn't happen, we are deprived of our need to achieve, and it is destructive to our self-worth. Disturbances, imbalances, and disharmony in our relationship with other people, especially family members, has a devastating effect on us.

Our Sensual Dimension

We have beautiful sensory channels. Some people's channels don't work very well because of frank physical impairment of the sensory organs. For people not so affected, the sensory channels still might not work well. It is easy for all of us to distort, through expectation or past experience, what is happening in the present. Furthermore, our sensory channels have been made suspicious by early admonitions of "don't look," "don't touch," "don't listen," and the like. As a result, our intake channels are working only part-time, and then only partially. In this situation, present conditions and people are not taken in as they really are. Instead, they are taken in as how they should be, how they were, or how they will be. This clearly leads to imbalances.

Our Emotional Dimension

From what I can gather from my experience, literature and my learned friends, the right brain (together with our nervous and glandular systems) is the vehicle by which we monitor and experience our feelings. Feelings are the vehicle by which we experience life's happenings. They are the "juice" that gives color and texture and tone to our lives. It is in this area that human beings (in the interest of being acceptable) ignore, deny, distort, or project their feelings. This, in turn, distorts their perceptions and inhibits their creativity and competence. All of this contributes to their state of poor being. A further result is that this works out in such a way that people deny themselves the love and respect that they so strongly desire from others.

Most of us in Western culture have been brought up to censor certain feelings, like anger, frustration, love (except with the "right" persons), and fear. The likely result is that then we ignore ("I didn't notice..."), deny (It didn't happen..."), distort ("It is something else..."), or project ("It is your fault... ") our feelings. Feelings are energy, and when they are not acknowledged, as they are, they take another form. The energy doesn't go away just because feelings are not acknowledged. Instead, it often resurfaces in destructive forms, which may be physical (as in illness), intellectual (as in thought disturbances or limitations), or emotional (as in nervous or crazy). Relationship disturbances are bound to follow. Negative inroads into self-esteem also result when this becomes a main way of being. The way is then created for the natural reinforcement of the negative conditions, whether they are manifested on a personal or interactional level.

Our Intellectual Dimension

Our intellectual part stems largely from the left brain, the home of logic. It is the thinking part of ourselves. Here is where we draw conclusions, make rules, accept beliefs, and become "scholarly." It is a marvelous vehicle for processing factual data. When it acknowledges the right brain as an equal partner, it can create all kinds of excitement, discovery and curiosity for its owner.

Unfortunately, Western culture has somehow given a much higher status to the left brain, and, in all fields where knowledge and scholarship is to be uppermost—science, medicine, technology, etc.—the right brain has been downgraded, with a result that we starve ourselves. Only people in the arts are esteemed for their right brain work.

On the whole, women have been denied the use of their left brain, and have tried to get it through men. Men, on the other hand, have been denied the use of their right brain, and have tried to get it through women. This has made us a culture of "half wits," and many disturbances in male-female relationships can be traced to this.

This seems to be changing. My hunch is that we are entering a period where we know that human beings have to have, acknowledge and use both right and left brain, and to honor both the thinking and feeling parts of themselves so that we can become "whole wits."

Our Physical Dimension

Our bodies are miracles. Who could have dreamed up such marvels and then made them work? For the most part, we have been taught to ignore our bodies, except when they are dirty, sick, too fat or too lean, or not the right size or shape. The idea of loving, appreciating, understanding and communicating with our bodies is just beginning.

When one hates, ignores or takes for granted one's body, imbalances and disharmonies result, which can show up in different manifestations affecting the body, feelings, thoughts and actions.

Having all these eight levels makes us a tapestry of parts, each part influencing and being influenced by others. These eight levels are the ones that are apparent to me now. Others are bound to be discovered.

Until recently, these various levels have been treated as separate entities, and the care of each has resided with a specialist. Often these specialists had little or no understanding or appreciation of how that part was related to the other parts. We put our bodies in the hands of physicians, our brains with educators, our feelings with psychotherapists, our souls with the

clergy, and the rest in a no man's land. In any given human being at any point in time, there is a dynamic interplay between all
eight levels. It would be as if there were a formula:

A (body) + B (brain) +C (emotions) + D (senses) + E (interactions)
+ F (nutrition) + G (context) + H (soul) = S (self).

All parts do add up to a self, although the self is more than
the sum of the parts. Still, each part can be studied separately.
But the truth remains that each of us is a system. While we can
talk about each part separately, they function together, just like
any system. Just like a family.

What we have now—the interrelationship between eight levels
—presents a very complicated picture for the therapist and family members to understand. Yet to truly understand what is going on, I think we need to start thinking and acting with this
kind of consciousness. As for me as a therapist, I look at what a
symptom in a system is saying about imbalances and difficulties
within these levels. I look at the rules of the individual or family
system, the values and information used by the person or family,
to help me understand what is stuck, undeveloped, prohibited,
or ignored.

I have a very oversimplified definition of a system. Briefly
stated, I see a system as a set of actions, reactions, and interactions among a set of essential variables that develop an order
and a sequence to accomplish an outcome. When I use the word
"family," I mean all the family forms, natural, blended, one-
parent, extended and communal. They all have basically the
same components.

Applied to a family, the essential ingredients are the adults
and the children in that family. One jointly held, explicit goal is
that the adults will steer the children in a course for successful
adulthood. The second, more implicit, goal is that each member
of the family will have satisfaction while this process is going on.

How parents arrange for coping with change, growth needs,
physical, mental, emotional and sexual growth needs, developing
and using power, intimacy, privacy, competency, achievement
and successful social relationships will result largely from the
rules of the system these parents have created.

I believe that such a system is based on what the adults, who
are in charge of the family, bring from their past experiences,

their hopes, knowledge, information and values. This is woven together through their self-esteem, communication, emotional rules, and survival vulnerabilities. The basic part of this is how the couple blends, dovetails or conflicts in their respective ways of dealing with each other.

I hasten to add that, as far as I can see, all parents do the best they can. Their best is dependent, of course, on what they have learned and how they feel about themselves. They are not to be blamed. Their behavior is a natural consequence of what they have learned. They need to be understood, made aware of themselves, and educated about how to be more fully human. When one studies at least three generations of a family, one can see in a crystal clear way the results of learning and degrees of self-esteem.

In an elementary way, I see that systems are generally of two basic kinds: open and closed. Closed systems in families seem to operate on a set of rigid, fixed rules that are applied to a given context regardless of how the rules fit. These systems have weak, distorted and rigid relationships with the outside world. An over-simplified example of this rule would be setting one's carburetor at a fixed point for oxygen intake and considering it fixed for all altitudes. Sayings like, "once a child, always a child," or "thirty five is the best age, so we must keep it that way," or "once sick, always sick" are also illustrative of the point.

A closed system is dominated by power, neurotic dependency, obedience, deprivation, conformity and guilt. It cannot allow any changes, for changes will upset the balance. People hang on to this balance because they are afraid. They seem to have a fantasy that a catastrophe resulting in total destruction will follow if change is permitted. This, of course, varies in degrees with different families. I made up an old saying: "What one knows, as uncomfortable as it may be, is more secure to many people than risking the perils of the unknown." This is what I call resistance. To make change we always have to risk the unknown.

The result of closed systems is that their members are kept ignorant, limited, and ruled through fear, punishment, guilt and dominance. A closed system has to break down over time because one or more persons comes to the end of their coping ability. When this happens, someone develops symptoms.

An open system features choice and flexibility. It even has the freedom to be closed for a while if that fits. The key to a healthy and open system seems to be the ability to change with a changing context, and to acknowledge that fact. It also allows full freedom for, and acceptance of, the full expression of hopes, fears, loves, angers, frustrations, stimulations and mistakes. In other words, the full range of what we know as human beings can be present without threat. The open system encourages the conscious development of self-worth, congruent communication, and is directed by human guidelines.

There are, of course, varying degrees of open and closed, because we are all human beings and are not perfect.

All systems in families are for the protection and management of their members. In closed systems, because they are managed largely by fear, the resources are experienced as limited and finite. People in closed systems live in a hostile world where love is counted in dollars, conditions, power and status. In open systems, managed by love and understanding, resources are seen as ever present possibilities. People live in full humanness with confidence, humor, realness and flexibility. Problems are treated as challenges to be coped with rather than as things to be defeated by. Part of that is seeking help when it is needed.

So what happens when a member of a system has trouble? (A bad boy or girl was never born. Only beings with potentials are born.) Something in that human being has to be denied, projected, ignored or distorted for him or her to become some kind of bad, sick, stupid or crazy boy or girl, man or woman. The answer to just how this happens is easy for me to explain, but very difficult to change.

This person is simply the outcome of all the transactions, both intentional and unconscious, that occurred between the child and himself and the other family members—especially the adults, who have had in their hands the power over his or her psychological life and death from the time of conception until the present. All infants are necessarily a captive audience for the beliefs of their parents and the society of which they are a part.

Human beings seem willing to pay whatever price is necessary to feel loved, to belong, to make sense, and to feel as if they matter, even if the price exacted doesn't really accomplish that. The self is willing to adapt to almost anything to try to get those things. This makes it possible for closed systems to continue as long as they do.

We have psychiatric nomenclature that gives names to the ways this kind of adaptation takes place, names like schizophrenic, manic depressive, etc. I remember that once it wasmore important to me to use those names in making psychiatric diagnoses than it was for me to understand the person.

Labels can be dangerous, especially if they mix up a description of a person's condition with his or her identity. Once given, such labels can form a new identity for that person, and can continue to reinforce the existence of that identity "the sick one," "the crazy one," "the little one," etc.

Diagnosis in the past has been, in effect, often a subtle or blatant blame process instead of an exploration horizontally and vertically in the person's life. Diagnosis, being pathology oriented, has dealt with the symptom.

But when we look at a symptom in light of it being an effort to adapt, we can understand better how to search for the meaning of the symptom. People with symptoms are trying to accomplish survival in what they perceive to be an alien, hostile, toxic system—and to give meaning to life. Usually the person feels helpless to change things, within or without, and may even try to struggle with it as being part of their fate.

Another way of looking at a person with symptoms is to see that they are starving to death. If I feel starved on any level, to the point of extinction, and I consider myself resourceless, I will grab at anything that promises nurturing where I am starving. This could mean: I would kill, steal, mutilate myself, assault others, cheat, etc. To some people meeting their starvation needs in those ways is inconceivable, so they resort to other ways such as drugs, alcohol, physical or mental illness, that can serve to disengage the hunger from their consciousness. In other situations, they see themselves as so without resources and meaning that they resort to suicide.

For me, the symptom is analogous to a warning light that appears on the dashboard of a car. The light, when lit, says the system required to run the car is in some form of depletion, disharmony, injury or impairment. One part, or a combination of parts, may be breaking down. If any one part breaks down, the whole system is affected. Just as in the family.

I see the family and the individual in the same way. My emphasis is on understanding the message of the light, and then on searching for ways that family members deplete, block, or injure themselves and each other. My treatment direction is to release and redirect that blocked up energy, which means I deal with their self-esteem, communication, and rules for being human as these relate to the eight levels of self.

My emphasis now is on developing and releasing health on all levels. When that is achieved, the symptom no longer is necessary and withers away from disuse. I find that family rules can be changed to human guides that can support human health, growth, happiness and love. This means a harmonious interplay between all levels—within oneself and between self and other members of the family.

If therapy is understood as a vehicle for releasing health and for making room for harmony, then therapy is a very acceptable way of coming to a new relationship with the self, so that the self can live fully, using the self's intellectual, emotional, physical, social, sensual, contextual, interactional, nutritional and spiritual resources. It is also a way for selves to use those resources between themselves. Maybe in the future, we will pay more attention to what it means to be fully human. It could become just as important to learn this as learning to read is now. Therapy would have a very different face then.

For now, one role of therapy is to look at the roots of behavior. It seems to me that the roots of all current behavior began as a specific response to a specific situation at an earlier moment in time. When that response occurred within a cluster of stress and was accompanied by a survival need, it began to form a new definition of that person. Once the new definition started, it became easy to reinforce. What we see in the present is that new entity. Gradually, over time, that once new definition became an identity, and a whole new set of responses were set in action.

What is often difficult for the therapist is to see the potential behind the symptom, because the effect of the symptom is so strong. Looking at any current behavior within the perspective of health and potential helps me to see that what I watch happening before my eyes can be understood. In other words, the psychopathology gets demystified. If I know about an event, and then know how that event was perceived, coped with and integrated, I can understand how similar subsequent behaviors have come about.

It has seemed clear to me for some time that the stated content problem was not the place to start with any symptom. It is the coping with the problem that is the problem. That is a process. I noticed that so many problems that people found devastating were events that are faced by many human beings. The difference between people who deal with their problems and those who are devastated by them is the coping process. I see that process as a function of degrees of self-esteem. Valuing oneself is also one key to health. Without high self-esteem we are vulnerable to all kinds of erosion of ourselves.

Despite what I and other therapists have written, we really know very little about health. Our attention has been so much on ill health. The lack of illness is not the same as health; no more than the lack of war is the same as peace.

In the past, many therapists looked at using strength as a basis on which to build as being simple minded or superficial. I feel that working on pathology is like beating a dead horse. There is no life there. I don't believe that we have much to show for the uncountable hours spent in the aggregate by all the people helpers in the world who have approached therapy from a pathological orientation.

In these days of holistic-health thinking, biofeedback, visual imagery and right/left brain integration, we can no longer see or behave as we did. I have seen over time the real advantages of looking at things from a health-oriented perspective.

For example, I have seen a group of people (twenty families) for a solid week, once each year for six years now. People have been born, come into adolescence, left home, gone to school, married, divorced, re-married, retired, and died. All of these were transitions that could have become psychiatric crises for these people. Instead, they were treated as normal life occurrences that heralded a change in the current situation; and they were treated as challenges, not crises.

Using oneself as a therapist is an awesome task. To be equal to that task, one needs to continue to develop one's humanness and maturity. We are dealing with people's lives. In my mind, learning to be a therapist is not like learning to be a plumber. Plumbers can usually settle for techniques. Therapists need to do more. You don't have to love a pipe to fix it. Whatever techniques, philosophy or school of family therapy we belong to, whatever we actually do, has to be funneled through ourselves as people.

In my teaching, I focus in depth on the personhood of the therapist. We are people dealing with people. We need to be able to understand and love ourselves, to be able to look, listen, touch and understand those we see. We need to be able to create the conditions by which we can be looked at, listened to, touched and understood.

The problem with techniques is that they can be used as cookie cutters—regardless of the size, consistency or texture of the dough. In the beginning, I suppose we all have to use cookie cutters to some degree. Later, we need to learn to be more relevant and expanded in the variety of the things we do and in the discreet use of techniques.

Recently, I filled out a questionnaire for family therapists to ascertain their style of therapy. I found myself saying "yes" to almost all the techniques. Yet, none of them represents me at every point with every person and family. I treat what I learned about psychopathology as information to use when it fits. It is not a matter of throwing it away, but of putting it in a new context. For me, the knowledge about how to change a flat tire will not teach me much about driving. I need both kinds of skills. I can't make one kind of learning responsible for the other. Psychopathology gives us information about pathology. It doesn't give us information about health. We need to know about and use both.

Techniques, though, are always of special concern. "What do you do?" or "How should I do this?" are questions very often asked of me. For me, a technique is a course of action taken at a specific moment in time to achieve a desired result. I have thousands of them. They are selected to meet a specific need with a person or a group of persons at a moment in time. If I don't have what I need, I invent it.

As of today, most leading family therapists would agree on how a family system with a symptomatic member operates. There is, however, considerable variation in ways of approaching it. Each therapist has emphasized different aspects. Many specialize in specific populations. It is clear that what the therapist emphasizes and utilizes has a lot to do with the personality and the beliefs she or he has about human beings.

Through what we have learned in family therapy, we have come to see individuals and families in a new light. It seems clear that the family is where the foundations for adulthood are formed, and also where the seeds for difficulty are formed.

What people are taught reflects the wider social group or society. If we want to change our society, we need to raise the levels of learning and individual consciousness concerning what it is to be more fully human.

People have always been searching, just as we do. And for all we have learned about human beings, there are still many mysteries.

Some of the things we learned that seemed fitting at the time of discovery turned out to be partially or completely discarded over time. For example, leeching is no longer considered a medical cure for fever. Some of the past discoveries were buds that had to be developed. And some were basic new discoveries. It will go on that way. It has been that way for me.

Any new information usually forces us to take a new look at present theory and practice and usually ends up in modifications and changes. The key is to be available to look at new information and be willing to try it on for size. I think this is very applicable to all people who act as experts on human beings. When one limits oneself in one's mind to having the "right way," and rejects all other things that do not fit that way, one becomes closed, and therefore dangerous.

At this point, I sit squarely on directing my therapy toward opening up awareness of the presence of human potentials in human beings. My efforts are also going toward the larger "families", such as our community, both national and political. The same ingredients apply as in the individual family. I see many others doing the same thing.

It seems we are just entering the era where we are discovering what a human being is and what it means to be fully human. All that I write now are just wee beginnings. To students five hundred years from now, it might be written that this was the time that feeble beginnings in this direction were being made. They will look at us as being in the prehuman times, much as we look back at people in the prehistoric times.

The seeds will continue to grow. One hundred years ago, few people could have foreseen the marvels of technology that have been created. Thirty years ago, no one applied the concept of system—known and applied in medicine and technology—to the family and our human organizations. We do now.

What the next thirty or one hundred years holds for us in the way of discoveries about human beings we do not know. Some of these discoveries will doubtless lead us to a deeper understanding about what human health is.

I, for one, look forward to that which will be discovered and created. In the meantime, while I am keeping an open mind, I work and live confidently with what I believe to be true.

References

Bandler, R., Grinder, J., Satir, V. (1975). *Changing with families: A book about further education for being human.* Palo Alto, CA: Science and Behavior Books, Inc.

Bateson, G., Jackson, D., Haley, J., & Weakland, J.H. (1956). Toward a theory of schizophrenia. *Behavioral Science,* 1(4), 251-264.

Satir, V. (1964, 1967). *Conjoint family therapy.* Palo Alto, CA: Science and Behavior Books, Inc.

Satir, V. (1970). *Self-Esteem.* Millbrae, CA: Celestial Arts.

Satir, V. (1972). *Peoplemaking.* Palo Alto, Science and Behavior Books, Inc.

Satir, V. (1976). *Making contact.* Millbrae, CA: Celestial Arts.

Satir, V. (1978). *Your many faces: First step to being loved.* Millbrae, CA: Celestial Arts.

Satir, V., Stachowiak, J., and Taschman, H. A. (1975). *Helping families to change.* New York, NY. Jason Aronson, Inc.

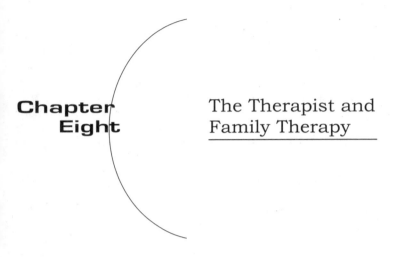

Chapter Eight

The Therapist and Family Therapy

Introduction by Sharon Blevins

People often marvel at the "magic" of Virginia Satir. How was she able to connect so effortlessly with people? How did she bring about deep, profound change in people's lives? Satir's "magic" was not a divine gift; rather, her unique and precious style is the direct result of her life-long educational journey. Her "magic" was deeply rooted in her belief in people's worth, her acknowledgment of the uniqueness of each individual, and her understanding of the importance of connection between people in relationship. This process began at an early age for Satir. As she nurtured her curiosity about relationships and became the self-proclaimed "detective" in her family of origin, Satir began carefully watching and curiously questioning the dynamics of her family's interactions. Because of her natural curiosity and her interest in interactions between people, Satir began to see the individual as unique, powerful, and—most of all—capable of bringing about change. In this article, Satir shares the model as she developed it throughout her lifetime. Beginning with her childhood detective work and moving through each major insight that built the Satir Model, Satir gives us a fascinating inside look at her own process of learning.

As Satir shares her development of the model, she unfolds her life-long journey of learning about people and relationships. Her original insights were gleaned from her own family of origin where she learned to connect with people by acknowledging their worth, building their trust, and inviting them to take personal risks. She became a companion on the journey toward transformation, encouraging people to become their own "detectives" and search inwardly for the resources needed to bring about hope and positive change. She focused on redirecting people internally to experience their feelings, which became a direct link to the building of self-esteem; this connection then allows the person to make different choices about his or her life. The process of building self-esteem though connecting with an inside feeling became the core of Satir's theory. Satir found that building self-esteem is essential before positive change can take place . She further developed her theory based on this discovery.

Satir believed " ... that the right brain is linked to the experience of the senses ... and, thus directly to the development of self-esteem." Her work with people involved connecting their minds, bodies, and feelings as a means to bring about change. She observed people's body language and found that many people repressed and denied their true feelings, which then somatized into a variety of physical ailments: back problems, intestinal problems, hypertension, asthma, skin rashes, diabetes, bed-wetting, etc. Satir believed that the body is linked to the senses and the memories that people carry. She developed the Communication Stances as a way for people to activate their right brain and safely experience their feelings about their past experiences. The experience of connecting the mind, body and feelings became a powerful means to building self-esteem, healing emotional wounds, and bringing about positive change. Current research today validates Satir's early beliefs about the connection between the mind, body and feelings. Psychoneuroimmunology (PNI), which studies the measurable interactions between people's beliefs, their behaviors, their brain function, and their immune systems, is researching and finding that people's beliefs and the repression of feelings are directly linked to physical ailments that people develop.

Today our world is busier than ever before. Our hectic lives can offer little time for self-reflection or connection to others, which can result in feelings of isolation and immobility in life. Satir's profound insights offer us a different way of living in the midst of our busy lives. Her work offers hope to people seeking to change their lives and the lives of others. Satir's "magic" is about touching an individual's inner world with acceptance, acknowledgment, and hope, thus bringing about the possibility of change and new life. Now, through her teachings, Satir's "magic" has been transformed *into a working model used around the world to bring hope and positive change to those who live in darkness.*

■ ■ ■

Most of what I am presenting in this chapter is concerned with how I learned, and am still learning, to see. I am a "homemade" family therapist in the sense that I have had no formal training in family therapy. I was, instead, one of the unorthodox people who, 29 years ago, stumbled onto the possibilities of working with the family as a treatment unit, and went from there. I was trained initially as a teacher, and then as a psychiatric social worker in a mainly psychoanalytic context.

My subsequent work with families illuminated many of the clinical concepts I had learned in my professional training. However, there were many more that I gradually had to discard.

I have chosen to write this chapter essentially as a personal chronicle of my journey of seeing and relating to people in need.

Definition

I feel the name *process model* fits how I see what I do. This model is one in which the therapist and the family join forces to promote wellness.

The heart of the model consists of all those interactions and transactions translated into methods and procedures that move the individuals in the family, and the family system, from a symptomatic base toward one of wellness.

In my view, all systems are balanced. The question is: What price does each part of the system pay to keep it so? The rules that govern a family system are derived from the ways parents maintain self-esteem and, in turn, form the context within which the children grow and develop their self-esteem. Communication and self-worth are the basic components.

Assumptions

I start with the assumption that any symptom signals a blockage in growth and has a survival connection to a system—which requires blockage and distortion of growth in some form in all of its members—to keep its balance. The form differs in each individual and in each family, but the essence is the same.

A further assumption is that human beings have all the resources that they need to flourish. My therapeutic process is to aid them to gain access to their nourishing potentials and to learn how to use them. This is what creates a growth-producing system.

I use eight levels of access: physical, intellectual, emotional, sensual, interactional, contextual, nutritional and spiritual. The symptom gives me a starting point, much like a point on a map, which shows where blockages are. And it gives me clues to aid in finding and releasing the distorted, ignored, denied, projected, unnourished and untapped parts of persons so that they can cope functionally, healthily, and joyously.

A third assumption is that everyone and everything is impacted by, and impacts, everyone and everything else. Therefore, there can be no blame—only multiple stimuli and multiple effects. This is a fundamental systems concept. An early step in intervention is to make this system pattern visible, felt and understood. *Sculpting* is one method I developed to make this possible. This is a method of having people take physical postures, together with components of distance and closeness, which show their communication and relationship patterns.

Sculpting involves having all the people present, in spirit, if not in body, who impact one another. This may include, in addition to the nuclear family, the family of origin (grandparents and in-laws), significant others, household help, and pets. When families are blended, this also includes, in a fitting way and at the relevant time, ex-spouses. I work a lot with families and in groups. I can then use role players for the absent ones. In the office situation, I use empty chairs or work with visualizations, and sometimes role playing, using family members.

I act upon a fourth assumption, namely that (a) therapy is a process that takes place between persons and is aimed at accomplishing positive change, and (b) the therapist can be expected to be the leader in initiating and teaching a health-promoting process in the family. The therapist is not, however, in charge of the persons involved. The love, trust, and risk context that I develop are the means by which I help people to take the risks they need to take to start taking charge of themselves. As long as I take charge of a person, relatively little gets accomplished. The process I initiate is heavily weighted toward each member of the family becoming as whole as possible.

Historical Development of the Model Precursors

Long before I had professional training, I had to work my way up from being a child. When I was 5, I decided to become a children's detective on parents. There was so much that went on between my parents that made little or no sense to me. Making sense of things around me, feeling loved, and being competent were my paramount concerns. I did feel love, and felt I was competent, but making sense of all the contradictions, deletions and distortions I observed—both in my parents' relationship and among people outside in the world—was heart-rending and confusion-making to me. Sometimes these situations raised questions about my being loved, but mostly they affected my ability to predict, to see clearly, and to develop my total being.

Becoming a detective meant becoming an observer. Naturally, I put all the clues I had together to make the best wholeness I could. This was my reality. The human brain has to make sense of what goes on, even if it is nonsense. In those days, faithful to the format of detective stories, I needed to find out who was the "bad guy," to catch him/her, then punish him/her, and, subsequently, to try to bring about reform. Sometimes the culprit would be me, or one or both of my parents.

I was curious about everything, including those things I was "too young for," or that "weren't for girls." Accordingly, I developed a capacity for storing secrets, presumably without giving any clues. I loved school, was an insatiable reader, and got "very high" on ideas, particularly on knowing how things work, and what they are made of.

Every once in a while, I would put words to some of my observations, and would tell my parents about their behavior. I got varying reactions: dismay, shame, amusement, surprise or sometimes silence. I never knew what went into each variation. The same oral observation would get different reactions from each parent at different times. My handling of this was to make jokes, behave as if I were deaf and dumb, and, many times, to behave as though I had my attention elsewhere. I had twin brothers, 18 months younger than myself, who were quite useful in this regard.

Somewhere there was a whole world (inside human beings) that I meant to investigate. I felt a deep connection with all children. They were my troops. They were my focus. I was nearly 30 years old before it dawned on me that all adults were just children grown big. If they hadn't learned anything more since childhood, they would still be doing childish things. This bit of insight helped me to understand adults a lot better.

The natural thing for me "when I grew up" was to be a teacher of grade school children. My education to become a teacher taught me about how children learn (learning theory), and especially about appreciation and respect for the human capacity, and some inklings about the influence of parents on children. I was fortunate to have a group of very gifted and very human instructors who inspired me to continue to observe, and listen and draw my own conclusions. At this point, I enlarged my scope of understanding. These instructors helped me to keep a nonjudgmental attitude toward human beings. I felt like a humanistic scientist in a laboratory of children's lives.

I wanted to be a "real live" expert on children instead of an "armchair expert," so I arranged my six years of teaching experience in five different schools, which were in different economic and social groups in widely scattered geographical areas. Among these were physically and mentally handicapped, gifted, racially different, and so-called "average" children.

When I stared teaching, it seemed natural to me that, if I wanted to help children, I needed to know their parents. So I proceeded to visit a different child's home every evening after school. This home visitation program helped me develop strong bonds with over 200 families during those 6 years.

Armed with little more than intellectual understanding from my undergraduate training, my observations became more focused. Through my contact with individual family members, I soon began to put two and two together. For example, there was one youngster who seemed listless and uninterested in school and who looked like he needed help. When I got to know the family, I found that they were night owls. Everyone else could sleep late in the morning, but this lad had to get up early. I arranged a nap time for him and shared the situation with the family, who then used their resources to help out. I know now that my nonjudgmental and human feelings drew them to helping me so I could help them. With their help I was a better teacher to this little boy, and he was a better student with all of us helping.

Another lad came to school very dirty and hungry. When I investigated, I found out that his father went on binges. At night he would lock his son out. I didn't "cure his alcoholism," but we were able to work it out so that the child was not locked out any more.

Another child was always scratching and itching. It turned out that she had lice. Because of my relationship with the family, we could take the steps that would cure the problem without creating stigma and embarrassment.

A mother of another young boy, then 10, told me that the boy had been tied to a tree when he was 5, and genitally abused by older boys. The effect was that he often had lapses of consciousness. She asked me to protect him in woodshop so he would not injure himself while using the electric saw. He was passive and undersized. His mother told me she had looked for help everywhere and had found none. My first response was to join her in becoming her friend. Then, feeling her support, I agreed to do what I could, knowing absolutely nothing technically about what to do to help the boy, yet trusting that somehow I would find something.

My way in teaching children was to create an alive context, play games, do skits, paint ideas—in short, to do anything to touch their excitement and turn them on to learning. In the case of the 10 year old boy, I initiated a project of making puppets, and then produced a fairy tale. I selected one that had a terrible "bad guy," and a "marvelously pure savior." It ended up with the young, meek little boy who had been abused playing both parts. He would stand behind the puppet curtain where no one could see him act, and he would become the most ferocious bad guy, with a voice that got bigger and bigger. And he could be a most competent good guy. After about 50 showings (we took the show around town), this child had physically grown nearly 2 inches, and his lapses of consciousness were gone. He later became a successful member of his varsity team in college and, still later, a successful professional person.

It was many years before I understood fully what had happened. What I was learning at this early stage was that:

1. Parents can be assets to their children if we know how to enlist their help.
2. If children have problems, something is going on in the family or has happened in the past that affects the child.

3. Difficult problems can be solved if we trust that they can, if we create a trusting atmosphere, and work at gaining access to the necessary human resources.

My detective work was giving me more pieces, but I still didn't understand about how they fit together. I knew that success had something to do with what goes on inside people as well as outside. I heard about something called social work, where one learns about people's insides. I made plans, after two years of teaching, to enter summer sessions; and four years later I entered as a full-time student. I then got caught up in the excitement of pathology, and essentially forgot what I had learned about the growing potential in people.

In graduate school, I learned about the world existing within people, and especially about something that I interpreted as drives, within ourselves, that become powerful factors in our behavior. Since these drives are out of our awareness, they are also out of our control, as well as our understanding. In social work school, I learned intellectually about these "pathological" parts. I learned also that to help someone necessitated having rapport and investigating feelings—really a new intellectual concept to me. All of this was very exciting.

Prior to and following my graduation, for about ten years, I worked with delinquent girls in a setting where I followed the same course I had in teaching school—that is, I attempted to get in touch with the girls' families. There were many who were listed as having either no parents at all, or mothers but no fathers. It seemed important to find out who, and where, their parents were. I played detective again, and discovered the whereabouts of most of the parents, some of whom were still living, and some who had already died. In the cases where the parents were dead, I took the girls to the cemetery. The search for the parents brought me in contact with the very, very ugly part of life facts—mental hospitals, dirty rooming houses, death under horrible circumstances, poverty, neglect, morgues and hospitals. Regardless of all that, I had hope for everyone. I set about trying to reach the "little self-worths" in each person, which by now I knew, without any question, were present. Most of the time I succeeded in not only helping girls, but their parents as well. I could enlist their help in their own behalf, as well as that of their children.

I had developed a profound and unshakable belief that each human can grow. After 42 years, that belief is stronger than ever.

My search is to learn how to touch it and show it to people so they can use it for themselves. That was, and still remains, the primary goal in my work. It means a special tailoring for each situation. I came to learn, upon starting clinical work, that that kind of detective work was called "diagnosis." What I had learned about awakening the hope in people was called "developing motivations."

In clinical work, I learned the psychiatric nomenclature. I could "diagnose" with confidence. This meant I was "professional." It enabled me to talk "professionally." It enabled me to talk "professionally" with my colleagues ("professional" jargonese), as well as to write impressive reports. It, however, did not always result in helping people very much.

Frequently, I felt that I was doing some kind of "name calling" when I diagnosed. My profession seemed to require it. The things in my clinical work that I was trained to look at were all negative. My sense told me that, somewhere, there had to be something positive. (I certainly wasn't putting anything into anyone.)   It reached a point where I got a twinge every time I wrote a clinical diagnosis. It gradually dawned on me that it was because I was looking at only part of the picture. I began to understand why I felt so overwhelmed by what I was looking at. I could not treat someone whom I labeled "paranoid" or "schizophrenic"; I could, however, help someone who felt empty and useless. It was the same person, but by viewing that person as a person instead of a category, I could relate, and things would happen.

I learned nothing positive about other family members in my clinical work. At best, they were looked upon as dubious helpers; at worst, enemies. I had laid aside the experience I had gained as a teacher because then I was working with "healthy kids." Now, I was a clinician and was looking at sick people and their pathology. I was fast becoming a "mental-ill-health" specialist.

Because I needed personal help, and because it was also felt to be beneficial professionally, I sought out the help of a classical psychoanalyst. I gained something, but the basic difficulty was never touched as I proceeded to make the same mistakes all over again. I knew there had to be something more. That search for something more put me in no-man's land.

In 1951, at the urging of a close psychiatric friend, I went into private practice. Now I was on the firing line. Being nonmedical, there was no liability insurance nor third-party payments for me.

If I were to survive financially, I needed to get results; and if I were to survive professionally, I had to do it without making people worse or, even more scary, having my patients threaten or commit suicide. To compound the situation, the people who initially found their way to me were either people whom no one else would touch or people who were "long-time alcoholics," "chronic schizophrenics," extremely dependent, or who had undergone treatment from others who had given up on them; they were all high risk.

Two things happened. First, knowing that all the classical treatment regimes had been tried, I realized that there was no point in my repeating them. I laid aside, for the time being, my "clinical professional self," and went back to my detective work of former years, which brought me back to observing, listening and looking for health. Then one day, the second thing happened. After I had worked for six months successfully with a young girl who had been labeled "an ambulatory schizophrenic," I was called by her mother who threatened to sue me for alienation of affection. That day, somehow, I heard two messages in her statement—a plea in her voice tone, and a threat in her words. I responded to the plea and invited her in. To my surprise, she agreed. (I had been taught that she wasn't supposed to do that.) When she came to join her daughter, lo and behold, the daughter was back at square one. When I got over my shock, I again began to observe, and saw what I later came to know as the nonverbal cueing system, part of the double-level message phenomenon. This was the beginning of my communication theory. It became clear that words were one thing, and that body language was something else.

Eventually, it occurred to me that the mother might have a husband and the girl, a father. I inquired. (In child guidance practice, fathers were not included. Women had charge of the family.) There was a father and he was still living. I extended an invitation to the wife and daughter to have the husband-father join. They agreed, and he came. Now I was privy to a new phenomenon. Mother and daughter had been doing well. With father's coming, a very different drama unfolded. I was now dealing with what I later came to know as the *primary survival triad*. This is now a conceptual cornerstone of my work. We all start life in a triad. The way this primary triad is lived is what gives us our identity. Somehow it had been assumed, and seemed to be take for granted everywhere, that a triad had to be potentially destructive. The best one could hope for was to manipulate it so that it was benevolent rather than malevolent. I now know that in successful family therapy, the outcome rests on accomplishing a nourishing triad.

I now know that this triad is the source of the destructive or constructive messages children receive. Thinking back to my brothers and sisters, I wondered one day whether there were other children in the family. Upon inquiring, I found that there was a brother—who turned out to be the "good guy" with his sister being the "sick one." I was now in touch with what later I understood to be the family system; I was to see this particular form many times in the future.

I was observing a new phenomenon and, being the detective that I am, I kept watching and listening, hoping to find some connection with previous experience. I extended the learning I gained with this family to all my other patients. I eventually worked with people who were delinquent, alcoholic, psychotic, or handicapped physically or mentally. I began to see different variations of the same theme. In the interest of survival, people were conforming to something that worked against them. A child would lie so mother would continue to love her; people would say "yes" when they felt "no," and so forth.

During this period, I had a great deal of experience with people who were somaticizing. Here I learned about the powerful link between body, mind and feeling. The body is willing to accommodate itself to the most destructive directions issued by the mind. I began to see that the body said what the mouth denied, projected, ignored or repressed. I saw this manifested in back problems, gastro-intestinal disturbances, asthma, skin eruptions, diabetes, tuberculosis, propulsive vomiting, bed-wetting and other ailments. I also began to see that the body parts became a metaphor for psychological meaning.

It was while observing the body-mind-feeling phenomenon that I developed the communication stances that were later incorporated into literal *body postures* (placating, blaming, superreasonable, and irrelevant). Those stances gave a vivid picture of what was going on. When I put people into certain postures, I noticed that they developed much more awareness. I know now that the physical act of posturing, which I extended into sculpting, activated the right brain experience so people could feel their experience with minimal threat. They were experiencing themselves, instead of only hearing about themselves. Awareness could be developed.

There are now many body therapies. I believe the body records all the experiences one has. When the body is postured and sculpted, the old experience returns and has a chance for a new interpretation.

Once I began to get inklings that the body, mind and feelings formed a triad, I began to see that, if what one feels is not matched by what one says, the body responds as if it has been attacked. The outcome of this is physical dysfunction, accompanied by either disturbances of emotion or thought.

I learned that I could see this discrepancy in the way people communicated with one another. I watched for the discrepancy between verbal and nonverbal levels in communications. I began to see that all nonverbal messages were a statement of the Now. The verbal part could come from anywhere: past, present, or future. Often this verbal component reflected the "should" or the inhuman rules one had. The forms of discrepancy were manifest in:

1. *Inhibition*, what one felt but could not say.
2. *Repression*, what one felt but was unaware of, and only reacted to in another projection.
3. *Suppression*, what one consciously felt, but since it did not fit the rules, one denied its existence.
4. *Denial*, what one felt but ignored as unimportant.

Out of the clear blue in January 1955, I got a phone call from a man who was then a stranger to me, a Dr. Kalman Gyarfas. He was heading an innovative training program for psychiatric training, which was the forerunner of the Illinois State Psychiatric Institute, based in Chicago. Dr Gyarfas was interested in the family relationship between identified patients and their family members, and he asked me to become an instructor in family dynamics for the residents.

By now, I had completed four years of working with families. They numbered over 300. I had been busy working with exciting ideas and had been having good results. Now, to teach, I had to conceptualize what I had been doing. In doing this, I found out more clearly what I had been learning. Indeed, as I taught it, I also learned more about what I meant, and I became aware of the glaring gaps in my theoretical base.

Dealing with the psychiatric residents' experiences and their questions helped me greatly to fill in the holes and to clear up my fuzziness. New possibilities were revealed. All this training was done with state-hospital patients, who were a mixture of persons in both acute and chronic states.

Here, I formulated that what I was doing was using the interaction between family members to understand the meaning and the cause of the symptom. I saw how family members clued each other on levels that they were unaware of.

Over time, I saw the need for developing an overview to understand the process. I developed something called the *Family Life Fact Chronology,* which featured what happened, when, with whom, who went out, who came in, and other details. This was based largely on events and outcomes. I stayed away from the subjective emotional reactions. I put this chronology in a time frame so I could see the outcomes of family members coping over time.

This chronology started with the birth of the oldest grandparents, and succeeding events were brought up through time. (Since we live by time, I chronicled by time.) Generally, most case and medical histories chronicled only the negative events that had emotional or medical impact. In my chronology, I wanted to have a firmly documented background with which to look at the context in which the current situation existed. This tool became the backbone of another basic technique called *Family Reconstruction.* Family Reconstruction is now part of my therapeutic tool kit.

Previously, when I took histories, I would file separate pieces of information, such as "when I was 5, I had several accidents." In one place I might record "in 1936 my brother was born," and in other place, I might read that father "lost his job when I was young," or that "mother became depressed and was hospitalized." When I put all this into a specific time frame, it turned out: "When I was 5, I had several accidents; it was also 1936. Mother was hospitalized shortly after the birth of my brother, and father lost his job at the same time." That makes a clearer picture of the stresses involved. I also began to see that outbreaks of symptoms often occurred around a clustering of stress factors.

All these facts produced a context in which one could understand better the meaning of the symptom. Instead of isolating the facts, I put them in a time frame. Important new connections began to emerge. Patterns over generations became obvious. This also helped me to see people in the perspective of human life rather than only categories. Making a Family Life Fact Chronology became a requirement for those training with me. It aided them in coming to understand and appreciate the family as a context in which people lived, coped and struggled, as they responded to life events.

Sitting in my office reading a professional journal one day in 1956, I became absorbed in an article entitled "Toward a Theory of Schizophrenia," by Gregory Bateson, Don Jackson, Jay Haley, and John Weakland. I remember the thrill of reading that other therapists' work affirmed what I had been seeing in my work with families. While I had continued to have good relationships with my professional colleagues in Chicago, many of them later confided to me that what I was doing sounded freaky to them. Jackson and his associates were clearly supportive of what I was doing.

In the article, there was some information that helped me to understand better what I was doing and seeing, and some clues as to why it was working. I began combing the literature to provide a bibliography for the residents. I found a reference to Murray Bowen, Bob Dysinger, and Warren Brady, all MDs, who were engaged in research on schizophrenia that brought whole families to reside at the National Institute of Mental Health.

I immediately contacted Dr. Bowen. He graciously invited me to visit. He was probably as lonely as I was. At that time, working with families was unknown.

When I visited Dr. Bowen, I saw and heard so much that again validated what I had experienced and what I had conceptualized. Here was more support.

I continued my teaching of the residents for three years. Then, in 1958, for personal reasons, I move to California. Since my instructorship was only part-time, I continued my private practice. I regarded private practice as a kind of laboratory that gave me material to feed into my teaching. Then there came a significant turning point. Remembering "Toward a Theory of Schizophrenia," it was natural for me to contact Don Jackson when I moved to the San Francisco Bay area in California.

I had hardly begun to tell him about my work with families when he invited me to present my findings to his group at the Veterans Administration Hospital in Menlo Park. That group was composed of Gregory Bateson, John Weakland, Jay Haley, Bill Fry and a few others. That was February 19, 1959. Don then asked me to come to Palo Alto and help him, together with Dr. Jules Riskin, to open an institute. On March 19, one month later, the Mental Research Institute was opened. It was originally conceived of as an institute dedicated to researching the relationship of family members to each other, and how those relationships evolved into the health and illness of its members. The men involved agreed that family interaction seemed to behave like a system. Don Jackson and Gregory Bateson and their colleagues had studied one family in depth, in which there was one "schizophrenic" member, and they had been able to conceptualize the rules of that family system and to dramatize them in a simulated family which, when heard on tape, sounded authentic. One of the rules of science is that when you replicate your experience you have discovered a new truth. Jules, Don, and I succeeded in getting a good research grant.

After a few months, I was keenly aware that research was boring to me. I felt that I needed to develop a training program, and took it on as my next project. It was completed and opened to students in the fall of 1959. To the best of my knowledge, this was the first formal training program in family therapy. Actually, I was building on the experience I had had at the Illinois State Psychiatric Institute.

I developed a program which had three levels of training: Beginning—6 weeks, one evening weekly; Intermediate—twice monthly for 5 months; and Intensive—1 year, one day per week. I started with 12 brave souls, a mixture of all the disciplines: psychology, social work, and psychiatry. (In those days, family therapy was still freaky, and only genuine risk-takers applied.)

In 1964, at the suggestion of Gregory Bateson, I became acquainted with Eastern thought through Alan Watts and S. I. Hayakawa, a leader and student of general semantics. These contacts led to my discovering Esalen, a growth center in Big Sur, California, which had a profound effect on my professional thinking. Here I learned about sensory awareness, Gestalt therapy, transactional analysis, altered states of consciousness and the so-called "touchy-feely" experiences, encounters, body therapies and other nontraditional therapy modes. I found again that the relationship between how one sees things, and how one interprets what one sees, determines the direction one takes.

I used to ask my students to state their views about (1) how growth takes place, (2) how growth becomes distorted or repressed, and (3) how the normal growth process is restored or established. The first question is related to healthy development, the second to symptom development, and the third to so-called "treatment."

I found, in the main, that most professional training had been based on pathology being the center of attention, with health being a possible offshoot. Today I see the strivings for health as the center, with symptoms being a barrier or stumbling block to that health. In my clinical training, I was taught to focus on treating ill health, which, if properly done, would result in the absence of a symptom. There was an underlying assumption that the absence of ill health was the same as the presence of health. I found this to be no more true than that the absence of hair on the female face was the same as the presence of beauty in that face.

While at Esalen, I was exposed to the concept of the *affective domain,* an area of study in which Charlotte Selfer was one of the main teachers. This had to do with the senses, important in my work mostly through their dysfunction, but considered here in a different way.

I began to understand that seeing, hearing, and touching are experiences in themselves, and not confined to the objects they are related to. The experience of seeing, hearing, and touching— which, in turn, is related to feeling, thinking, and moving—is the essence of life. I learned that it is quite possible for a person to be so focused on what he or she is seeing that the experience of seeing is quite overlooked. For example, one may not be aware of smelling and tasting food, but only of eating. This is probably the case with people who overeat. I observed that it is possible to listen to the rhythm or lyrics of music without ever experiencing the music. I often hear people relate that they could wash their hands without ever having the sensation of touching. I began to learn how to help people extend their awareness of their sensual reactions, and watched their sense of self-worth expand.

It was sometime before I put together the ideas that the right brain is the center of our feeling self and is linked to the experience of the senses and that well-being is directly linked to the feeling of vitality and, thus, directly to the development of self-esteem.

The central core of my theory is self-esteem. I now clearly see that without a direct link to the experience of the senses, there would be little change in feeling. Consequently, there would be little change in self-esteem, and therefore little real, dependable change in behavior.

This, of course, is a far cry from looking at individuals, as I had been trained to do in my earlier clinical work, as masses of pathology. At this point I was approaching a holistic model, the glasses through which I look at human beings. Since we were all born little, our concept of ourselves is made up of all the interactions around us, about us, toward us. We develop our concepts as a result of a system.

Starting in June 1959, I was invited to consult and teach family therapy in different state hospitals in California. The request circle began to widen. I was invited to agencies for juvenile and family service in California. The mental hospitals in neighboring states invited me. This broadened to include the Army, Veterans Administration, and other. These requests have continued and now reach me from 14 foreign countries, with more on the way. In 1964, I published *Conjoint Family Therapy*.

What seemed to be happening to me was that I used my most up-to-date glasses to view my new experiences. I was fortunately able to change my glasses when I came upon new things. From this ability, I saw that growth was an ongoing process of sorting, adding on, and letting go of what no longer fit.

I feel as if I have been seeing layer after layer of a huge onion come into view. I realize that I will never live long enough to see all the layers that are there. I find myself going with what I have, and I am prepared to add that which fits and to let go of that which no longer fits.

I am compelled and impelled to understand the nature of life: what happens to stymie life, and what happens to transform it, what process makes it move and change, what factors nourish it, and what factors deplete and damage it. I saw therapy originally as concerning itself with that which damaged life, and finding ways to repair it. I now see therapy as an educational process for becoming more fully human. I put my energies and attention on what can be added to what is present. To explain it in an over-simplified way, I find that when one adds what is needed to one's life, that which one no longer needs disappears, including the symptom. I call this my concept of *transformation and atrophy*.

I pay attention to the damage, but with the emphasis on what will develop health, instead of trying to get rid of what is wrong. I have been trained as a human pathologist. I am now working as a "health developer," using the information of pathology to help me recognize trouble spots more or less in the same way that the driver or pilot uses the red indicator on a panel of a car or an airplane. It tells me that something needs attention.

Many questions present themselves: Does there have to be destruction in the human condition? Is it a precursor to developing strength? What are the best ways to restore health?

I started with individuals, then expanded to pairs (couples), and eventually to families. Now I work with groups of families, and also groups throughout the world.

At each of my turns in life new possibilities seem to exist. These take me more deeply into the nature of human existence and the meaning of life. Exploring altered states, spiritual planes, and cosmic connections seem to be natural next steps to take to further understanding of the nature of life. What we learn here may improve our day-to-day living experiences with ourselves, our intimates and our society.

Application

If I follow the philosophy I have just outlined, then family therapy is for everyone. I believe that any reader of this chapter will know that the elements of feeling, thought, and action are essential to each other and need to become a unified whole in each person's experience.

Family therapy is first a view about people. Everyone started in a family; therefore their present outlook reflects their early learnings in that family.

My view is that we are constantly trying to make a whole out of that which was unwhole in our growing up. When people have serious difficulties in their present, they are still trying to create wholeness or make up for their past. Even in the case of an individual or pair, this concept would be applicable.

Now that we know about systems, it makes sense to treat all the parts of the system. Thus, we treat the whole family. We learned a long time ago that, if we take out one part of the system, isolating it from the rest, we essentially make that part alien to the primary system: we create the phenomenon of rejection.

Furthermore, to have all the parts of the family physically present, we are able to create a support network for all people. For the most part, the family contains the resources, which when accessed and transformed, can heal the family. Just as in the untransformed state, these same resources were used to injure the family.

When we pluck out the offending part (identified patient) without reference to its related parts (other family members), we generally make matters worse, except in unusual circumstances. It was not so long ago that we believed that we needed to "cut off" the identified patient from his/her offending family and get him/her to "go it alone." We all know the destructive outcomes of that.

Depending upon the therapist's context, a person is referred, or comes voluntarily or involuntarily, having an obvious deficiency or behavior that is destructive to that person or to others. Commonly used names to identify such person are schizophrenic, depressed, suicidal, delinquent, criminal, alcoholic, drug abuser, slow learner, poor and unmotivated (public welfare people), relationship problem (child, marital, or family difficulties), and organ difficulties (asthma, skin problems, back and intestinal problems, and so forth). That person may be currently in a natural family, a one-parent family, a blended family (step, foster, adoptive), a communal or social family.

These are all avenues by which a therapist gets connected to her clients or patients. The initial unit can be the individual, a marital pair, parental-filial pair, a whole family, or a group. They can be called child, adolescent, adult, or geriatric. Whatever description is appropriate, you as therapist will be facing a person who has been a child and had gotten his knowledge through learning, no matter who or where he or she is.

I take whomever I can get at the onset of a therapy session, and depend on my skills to tap his or her health to bring in whoever else is needed. This usually works.

My first effort is to make real contact, and to demonstrate my feeling of the value of myself and each member of the family. This means shaking hands, a full focus of my attention on each person, a readiness to hear and listen, to be heard and listened to, to see and be seen, to touch and be touched. This process sets the tone and the context for the human contact among the people who will work together.

Metaphorically, and sometimes literally, I am offering myself as a temporary companion, taking the hand of each family member and creating learning situations in which we all can participate and benefit. This results in hope and trust that, in turn, permits the risk of doing and being something different. This, in turn, allows the flexibility for new growth to appear.

I trust the fact that if people truly feel valued, they will allow themselves to be more fully seen. I try to engage all persons as researchers of their own lives, with me originally being the senior researcher. This begins to change the blaming, which is so prevalent, into a puzzle for which we need to become first-rate detectives, students of life and experimenters.

For me, working with a family is like weaving a new tapestry: taking the threads from the used one, adding new ones, letting go of out-of-date ones and together creating a new design.

I often visualize in images and make frequent use of metaphors. I work from these images expressed directly, or used as a basis for indirectly making the new input. For example, I may make up a story about someone else that fits the family situation, but has different endings. Or, I might share an image and find out who, if anyone, shares this impression. As an example, I might say, "Right now I feel as though I were in a can of worms. Does anyone else feel that way?" Most of the time, some family members do.

As soon as possible, I make body postures of the current family communication patterns, and then sculptures of their movement. This would be the design of the old tapestry. People seem to find this method relatively unthreatening, and are quicker to identify their underlying feelings. Within this frame, these sharings become more a statement of what is, rather than indictments of others.

I see family therapy more as an experience, as a drama of real life, where many of the techniques of good theater are relevant. I encourage people to come to know their masks and also to be comfortable enough to look at what is underneath, so they expand their universe of choice.

I make use of literal ropes where I can show concretely the binds and pulls and demonstrate how ties can be experienced in many different ways.

In one sense, people present themselves as being made up only of bad stuff, blame, incompetencies and irrelevancies, which they protect through excuses, rationalizations, projections, denials and ignorance. I add the parts that are present but in the background, like their wish to belong, to feel and express their feelings without being judged, to matter, and to progress. I remind them of their successes, however small. This expands the perspective so that background becomes more prominent in the foreground.

People who become therapists, in whatever mode, need to remind themselves that they have chosen to deal with the destructive, ugly, and painful events in life, some of which can be "hard to stomach."

It is important to recognize that therapists are people, too, and may, in fact, have faced pain and ugliness in their own lives similar to that of the people they meet, whom they are trying to help. For me, it is helpful to acknowledge this first to myself, and then to others, when it seems appropriate. I can then be more able to separate me and my pain from those I am working with. I think it is important for family therapists to remember that the chances are high that all their ideals, their values, and their assumptions about family life all get thoroughly tested when working with other families. For example, we discover our own biases, "men should such and such," "women should. . . ," "children should. . . " Instead of judging what doesn't fit our bias, we must be more research-minded. Find out what is going on, and find out how the persons would like them to work better.

I find there is a Wise One in all of us, who, when we can have access to that one, can give us the direction we need to take. The challenge is to make contact with our Wise One. The Wise One in children is almost always up front and particularly manifested around the age of four. When adults, including therapists, listen and observe carefully, they can be guided by this wisdom. Fortunately, adults still have their 4-year-old self around somewhere, and under the appropriate circumstances, can reconnect with that wisdom.

One of the opportunities we have both to develop perspectives on ourselves and others is a sense of humor. If we look carefully at the human condition, we can certainly see both the tragedy and the comedy, often in the same event. What is the tragedy of today can, when properly viewed, become the comedy of tomorrow. I remember a woman who brought in her 8-year-old boy because he still ate with his fingers. When I asked her why she was concerned, her answer was that when he reached the age of 21, he would be in an important social gathering and would embarrass himself. I responded with mock incredulousness saying, "You mean in 13 years, he won't learn this!" We both laughed. Sixteen years later, this women called to tell me that all had turned out well. Her son was now a successful psychologist.

I want to make a few comments on technique. For me, a technique is something I use at a moment in time to make an intervention in order to allow something to happen. I have thousands of them in my resource basket, and am creating more each day.

Many of these were inspired by being exposed to systems theory (Gregory Bateson); interpersonal communications, psychoanalysis (Sigmund Freud); gestalt theory (Frederick S. Perls); transactional theory (Eric Berne); psychodrama (J. L. Moreno); psychosynthesis (Roberto Assigioli); body therapies (George Downing); life postural reintegration (Ida Rolf); bioenergetics (Alex Lowen); hypnosis (Milton Erickson); relaxation (autogenics); general semantics (S. I. Hayakawa); brain research (Karl Pribram); biofeedback (Swami Rami and Alyce and Elmer Green); transpersonal (Charles Tart); and now a whole range of New Age theorists and practitioners (Brugh Joy, Jack Schwarz, Rolling Thunder, Loma Govinda, Stan Kripner, Carl Rogers, Norman Sheeley, Carl and Stephanie Siminton, and business consultant Bob Tannenbaum). Most of these people are my contemporaries, and we were all part of an emerging new consciousness regarding humankind.

After writing all this, I am aware that there is no way I can even approximate a detailed ordering of concrete steps in the therapeutic process with families, or any other therapy, for that matter. Family therapists work out of their own centeredness, their life experience, and their professional skills and knowledge. Part of their centeredness relates to their attitude toward all life, and their commitment to use themselves to help the people they work with to discover the same for themselves.

I know I am limited by how and what I see, how I understand, what I know, and how I use that in the service of others. If I expand any of these parts, I expand my usefulness. I learned a long time ago that what I see, or know, or use doesn't represent all the possibilities for what could be seen, or known, or used. If I am open to new possibilities, I change from day to day and can successfully resist the idea of becoming orthodox, and thus limiting my usefulness to the people I serve. I could make my orthodoxy so prominent that the people would disappear.

Case Example

The following is an excerpt from a family interview that took place in a training session before 400 people. The family had been part of the seminar the previous day. Much had already been accomplished before I saw the family in this specific therapeutic family context.

The family was composed of Helen, the mother, 34; her mother, Mae, 65; her father, Bill, 67; and her two children, Maria, aged 10, and Darrell, aged 8. Russell, Helen's ex-husband, 35, was represented by a role player taken from the audience. (Names have been changed to protect confidentiality.)

The identified patient was the mother, Helen, who had been depressed and was living with her parents. Helen had been previously seen in individual therapy for a few sessions with the person who was referring the family to me. This was the first time these people had been seen together.

As the interview begins, we are seated in a circle. All six of us have microphones. The audience is supportive of this very delicate venture.

At the time of this interview, Helen and her two children, Maria and Darrell, had been living with her parents, Bill and Mae, since Helen's separation and divorce from Russell, her husband, 10 months previously.

Through the contact made the day before, I had developed good rapport with all of the family, including Helen's parents. Helen had told me in the morning of the day before that, although her parents were present, she doubted that they would get much out of it. At the end of that first day, she seemed genuinely surprised that her parents had participated so actively in the seminar, apparently learning a great deal. To her surprise, her father had initiated some discussion on previously closed topics.

I liked all the family members. I felt a mutual trust between us. They were interested, and demonstrated their hope for change.

Satir: Fine . . . OK. I don't know if your voice came through. I hope it did. So now that you come from this new space, what would you like to have happen for you, Helen, as a result of coming here?

Helen: Uh . . . the word that comes to mind is . . . realignment.

Satir: Realignment . . . putting something in order?

Helen: Uh-huh.

Satir: You want it in an order that it has been, or something different?

Helen: Uh . . . in the past two and a half years, since the end of my marriage, um . . . a lot of things blew up, lots of debris, lots of feelings, lots of changes in perception, lots of feelings. . . a lot of it very good . . . and there's a feeling for me of a culmination, of a birth or of a timeliness about this, and I really feel that it's a time to go forward and I feel this is an opportunity to kind of get things straight among the people I care most about.

Satir: Do you have any kind of pictures of something you would like to get straight, Helen?

Helen: Yes, a couple of things . . . uh . . . some in my relationship to my mom and dad, and some in relationship to my children. I would like . . . I've heard the term used . . . "permission," I guess is what is said . . . I would like for Darrell and Maria to have permission to feel free to ask any questions, to get very free with me and . . . about the divorce between their dad and me . . . and to just feel that they can come to me and I'll give them a direct answer and . . . I think . . . I'm concerned that I know they didn't feel that.

Satir: You want it so that . . . first, to Maria, because you can't talk to two people at once, so how about turning your chair so you can look at Maria. She may or may not have the questions you think, but at least you can start by telling her what you hope for. Can you do it even more . . . that's fine. It's good to have your shoes off sometimes.

Helen: Maria, honey, I would like for you to feel free to ask me any questions you have about Daddy and the fact that Mommy and Daddy are divorced and that he doesn't live in the same house with us anymore . . . and I would like to answer those . . . and I would like you to feel free to ask anything you want to know.

Satir: How are you feeling right now as you're sharing this with Maria and noticing her at this time?

Helen: Umm . . . I'm afraid of making her nervous. That's a lot to ask of her in front of a group, and it's not a new opportunity for her.

Satir: OK, now you want to turn your chair towards me a minute. We'll have a lot of chair turning here. What is your evidence that makes you think that Maria has questions she hasn't asked?

Helen: I'm more concerned with that with Darrell than with Maria.

Satir: All right, do you want to share this with Darrell, then? Turn your chair so you can direct your full attention to him . . . and maybe you might even want to go close enough, if he is willing, for you to take his hand while you talk to him . . . both of them . . . Now, how did that feel to you? Did you feel that Darrell was giving you his hands? All right. So, now at this moment . . . let's just be in touch with that. Maybe you could find out from Darrell how he felt about this invitation .

Helen: No . . . How do you feel about talking about that, honey? . . . asking questions. You can say absolutely anything here. *(Darrell nods his head "yes.")*

Darrell: I know.

Helen: OK

Satir: Now, do you believe Darrell? He says he knows he can ask any question.

Helen: I think he believes my words. I don't know that he feels that he can.

Satir: What's your evidence for feeling that Darrell is saying, "Yes, I can do that," and you don't think he can. What's your evidence? Averting his eyes. What are you feeling right this minute? . . . As I hear you want your child . . . and in this case, Darrell, to say whatever is on his mind. How do you feel right now, right here in this position with Darrell?

Helen: I feel ready.

Satir: OK

Helen: And I feel a lack of privacy for this.

Satir: You feel a lack of privacy. Does that mean you feel a little self-conscious at this moment?

Helen: Yes. Uh-huh.

Satir: Ok. Are you satisfied at this moment that Darrell has heard you?

Helen: Darrell . . .

Satir: Darrell.

Helen: Uh . . . I'd like to just ask him.

Satir: Well, that's open for you.

Helen: In fact, I would like . . . *(long pause)* . . . I would like to hear Darrell's feeling right now.

Satir: Why don't you talk to him.

Helen: Darrell, honey, I . . . I would like to know what you're feeling right now . . . if you can take a minute and . . .

Darrell: Nothing . . . *(long pause)*

(Previous information to Satir revealed mother still has unresolved issues about divorce.)

Satir: While you're over there, Helen, I would like to ask you, do you have any pieces that aren't connected for you about the divorce?
(This is an effort to supply a more living context for mother and son to deal with issues.)

Helen: Yes. Uh-huh.

Satir: OK. What's the name of the man?

Helen: Russell.

Satir: Russell. OK. Let's pick Russell out of the audience and sit him over here somewhere please. Would you pick him out?

Helen: Help me find him.

Satir: Well, you were the one who picked him out in the first place, so . . . *(laughter).*

Helen: I picked him yesterday too. Fred.

Satir: All right. If you can just find a chair somewhere, Fred, and then just come and sit here at the edge of the carpet to remind us all that you exist. How is that for you, what you just did Helen? You can turn your chair toward me a little bit.

Helen: That hurt a little bit.

Satir: Hurt?

Helen: Uh-huh.

Satir: Could you share what was gong on?

Helen: I want to cry already. I didn't think I could cry this soon *(crying)* . . . when you said, "You picked him . . ."

Satir: What happened then when I said, "You picked him"?

Helen: I remember getting this weakness . . . and then . . .

Satir: This weakness?

Helen: Uh-huh . . . and the innocence of that love . . .

Satir: And so something happened to you as you remembered that?

Helen: Very touching.

Satir: Very touching, Uh-huh . . . Does that still exist for you?

Helen: The innocence . . . the love?

Satir: Yeah.

Helen: Uh-huh . . . it's in a . . . yes, it's in ours, and I'd say it's in a package. I kind of put it that way.

Satir: Do you know how it happened that you and Russell separated? Because a few minutes ago, I heard you say to your children, "If you ask me, I will tell you." Do you know?

Helen: I know some of it.

Satir: What are your thoughts at this minute?
(very long pause)

Satir: What does it feel like right now?

Helen: Like being on the edge of a diving board.

Satir: Near the edge of a diving board?

Helen: Uh-huh. It feels precarious . . . but ready.

Satir: OK . . . and what does that readiness mean? . . . diving into what? . . . diving into an awareness of what happened to you and Russell?

Helen: Diving into trying to be as honest as I can about it . . . with me . . . and with Darrell and Maria.

Satir: How do you feel right now?

Helen: Contraction.

Satir: Contraction . . . when you came here today, was there something you wanted to do about that?

Helen: Yes. And I also have a task from Susan Arnold *(a therapist)* . . . which is to deal with having to take care of Daddy, which is the main thing . . . she didn't say much more than that.

Satir: OK. Well, now, Susan has set us a task . . . is that yours? Or are you just carrying out something for her?

Helen: When Susan and I were working I think that that was something, and I . . . and I . . . think that yesterday I began to deal with that.

Satir: . . . is it something?

Helen: . . . that there's a relief that . . . that has at least been opened up.

Satir: Let me see if I understand something.

Helen: Uh-huh.

Satir: . . . That as you think about Russell and what happened to you and Russell . . .

Helen: Uh-huh.

Satir: . . . a piece of what happened with you had something to do with when you learned to love your father? Or to feel his love for you? Something like that?

Helen: I think so.

Satir: And just a minute ago I reached out my hand and another hand came to mine. Did you see that?

Helen: Umm . . .

Satir: Do you see it now? When that happens right now, tell me what you feel.

Helen: I kind of want the other one.

Satir: Well, I noticed all I did was to reach out. Do you want to turn now toward him? *(Helen turns directly to Bill [father], sits in touching distance. Bill responds readily.)*
(background noise)

Satir: What's it like for you, right this minute, Helen? (pause) . . . to put words to what's there . . .

Helen: It feels like . . . uh . . . like I'm going to say good-bye . . . to being little . . . or, and uh . . . felt good to say that. Right afterwards it felt good.

Satir: OK . . . could you go a little further now, and I . . . hear you say, "Dad, I'd like to say good-bye to being your little girl." What do you want to say hello to? Could we move along to the next step?

Helen: I want to say hello to being a woman . . . not really . . .

Satir: Would that be to . . . be . . . a woman on a par with Bill, who happens to be your father?

Helen: Yeah. Uh-huh.

Satir: What are you feeling as you're letting that awareness come? That maybe there is a time now for a change in the way you view your father and how he views you? What does that feel like?

Helen: Gosh . . . you're nifty *(whispered)* . . . You're nifty! It feels Good!
(Helen looking directly at Bill while seated before him)
I like his eyes and I certainly . . .

Bill: Maybe you never looked before. *(laughter)*

Satir: How did you feel when Helen came out with, "You look nifty to me"? How did you feel, Bill, when that happened? Share it with her. Tell her.

Bill: Good.

Satir: What's it like for you right now, Mae, to watch your husband and your daughter do some different connecting?

Mae: Wonderful.

Satir: Want to say that to each of them?

Mae: It makes me feel wonderful.

Satir: Say it to them. Helen . . . and . . . What are you aware of right now?

Mae: I'm . . . aware of a veil lifting, and it's rather shocking to me . . . I'm aware of a sense of relief, and uhh . . .

Bill: Am I allowed to ask questions?

Satir: You may do anything you want.

Bill: What is it you want, sweetheart?

Helen: . . . from being little.

Bill: You mean that, uhh, I've been treating you like a little girl too long? I haven't allowed you to grow up?

Helen: . . . or I haven't insisted . . .

Bill: Huh?

Helen: I haven't insisted. I don't know, I don't care about that. I like this moment.

Satir: Good.

Mae: Me too.

Helen: *(laughs)* . . . 'bout time . . . No, I mean . . .

Satir: Go ahead, Mae.

Mae: Well, I was saying that after a year, our love for her . . .

Satir: Say it to her.

Mae: . . . for her and her sustenance, that's really kept us all going . . . we tried to help her with her problems.

Satir: Say it to her . . . we really tried to help you . . .

Mae: . . . to help you with your problems as much as we could . . . and you were always on our minds and our prayers.

Helen: I know that. I . . . and what I feel now . . . Darrell, do you want to come be with us? Come . . .

Satir: I'll take charge of this.

Helen: Thank you. I just, well . . . uhhh . . . I feel stronger all the time and more excitement and more joy about who I'm gonna become . . . and I don't want to be viewed as a problem any more or as a . . . a tragedy or a sadness.

Satir: Who are you talking to now?

Helen: To my mom and dad.

Satir: Think again, and ask who are you really talking to? You don't want to be a tragedy . . .

Helen: To me. To myself.

Mae: Well, Helen, I think in the last . . . can I say . . . the last six months if you will, you have grown much stronger, and I have felt that. And it has been a relief to me too.

Helen: You know, I'm glad to hear you say that because I think I felt, and one of the things I felt last night when we talked after your coming in the afternoon, was that maybe, to get attention or that . . . I had to be a problem or had to have a broken toilet or . . . *(laughter)* . . . and that's why yesterday when you came I felt a deep sense of relaxation, and another thing that you could come into my world that I was a little afraid to share with you for fear that it would cause separateness . . . and that in some ways I've blocked you out of things like . . . wanting to be a family therapist or my Peace Corps work and that . . . and I think it's just a vast underestimating of both of you . . . and, uh . . .

Bill: We weren't taken for granted, were we?

Helen: Yeah. *(laughs)*

Mae: . . . that's a surprise. . .

Satir: What are you feeling, Bill, about what Helen is saying right now? What are you feeling right in here? *(therapist touching center of Bill's abdomen)*

Bill: Well . . . just a little knotted up. No, I'm happy that . . . what she has said . . . that she felt she is growing stronger, which I, ahh . . .

Satir: Why don't you say that directly to her. You say that . . .

Bill: I feel that you're growing stronger, although I'm a little in doubt. Lately here we've been having so many telephone conversations, and that always puzzles me . . . ahh, I say, "I wonder what's wrong now." But we want you never to forget to call, because we want to be there when we're needed.

Satir: Could you start now talking about "I." You talk about "I" and Mae will talk about "I." That you'd like to be there. . . maybe Mae would like to too, but we'll let her talk for herself.

Bill: Gee, how will I start. *(laughter)*

Satir: Just use "I."

Bill: I don't know how to begin *(laughs)* . . . No, I want you to grow . . . I've been looking forward to you growing stronger and getting over these obstacles that, uh, you've had, and, uh, haloo . . .

Satir: What's happening to your knots right now, Bill?

Bill: They've disappeared.

Satir: At this moment, just at this moment, are you aware of any worry, small or big, which you have in relation to Helen?

Bill: No. No. Uh, she proved to me yesterday of her strength, her car didn't go *(Helen laughs)* . . . she had to . . .

Satir: Why don't you tell her that? "Your car didn't go," and I'll listen.

Bill: Your car didn't go , and you handled it immediately. You didn't go to pieces. You didn't even come to me and say, "Hey, Dad, what'll I do?" You took care of it yourself. And we had several times with it too. This made me real proud of you.

Satir: *(to Helen)* How does it feel in there, for you, now?

Helen: I feel about three different things. One is laughter. Uh. One is anger . . . at . . . the . . . lack of . . . I'm feeling, haven't you realized that I have taken care of myself before? and . . .

Bill: . . . not that positive . . .

Helen: And I'm thinking. While I felt the anger, then I was thinking . . . because you were so available, with no strings attached, that I used you rather than using me, and in the past 2 ½ years, I must have sensed that immediately, because, after, uh, Russell left, I couldn't and wouldn't come home. I couldn't go to visit. You could come see me, but I wouldn't go to you because I knew that . . . I had to grow up.

Bill: Yes, I understand that because one of the first things I said was, "You know you always have a home here . . . you and your children . . . "

Helen: And I said no.

Bill: That's right.

Helen: Uh-huh.

Bill: I even offered to send you on to graduate school if you wanted.

Helen: And I said no . . . I can do it . . . I'll do it . . .

Bill: . . . You'll go it alone.

Helen: Yeah.

Satir: *(to Mae)* What are you feeling right now as you're hearing your husband and your daughter again?

Mae: I'm . . . ah . . . feeling that . . . uh . . . Helen, that you have really grown in the last year, well . . . maybe part of it was my fault because . . . she's my daughter. . .

Satir: Well, why don't we just stop for a minute and let's see if you can take any credit for this. You said it was your fault, and I call that taking credit. I switch things around a little bit . . .

Mae: Well, maybe I did baby Helen a little bit . . .

Satir: Maybe you babied her a little, you say?

Mae: Ah, some, yes, but I still feel no. ' Course she hasn't been home since . . .

Satir: Talk directly to her.

Mae: . . . lived with us for a good many years since she went to college and got married, and . . . and . . . I feel right now, Helen, that you are stronger than when you were married.

Helen: So do I.

Mae: That's my feeling.

Satir: How do you feel now about how you might have been a little bit at fault?

Mae: Oh, I babied her too much maybe. She'd call on me and, sure, I'd do it. You know?

Satir: Did you do it to baby her?

Mae: No.

Satir: Why did you do it? Why did you do that?

Mae: 'Cause I loved her.

Satir: You did it 'cause you wanted to do something for her.

Mae: Right. Right. And I had the time to do it, so I did it . . . for ya.

Helen: And I want to go on record as saying it felt good . . . it feels good to grow up too.

Mae: Sure.

Helen: But it feels good to have you visit and know that you're going to make coffee in the morning. *(Mae laughs)*

Satir: Are you going to always have that? That when she comes to your house you're always going to make the coffee?

Mae: Sure, I'll make the coffee for her.

Satir: Don't you like to lay in bed sometimes?

Mae: I'm one that never did. *(laughter)*

Satir: I didn't ask you whether you did or not . . .

Bill: I make the coffee every morning. *(laughter)*

Satir: You're spoiling my story, Bill, just a minute. *(laughter)*

Mae: It's true.

Satir: So you get to stay in bed.

Mae: No, I don't really.

Satir: Well, are there two of you going around making coffee? *(laughter)*

Helen: If I'm there, she makes the coffee. If they're alone, he makes the coffee.

Mae: Or whoever gets up first makes the coffee, let's say.

Helen: But trying to beat either of them up is tricky.

Mae: No, wait.

Helen: Yes, it is.

Satir: Would you leave room when she comes to visit you, which will probably happen once or twice before the end comes, whatever that is, so that she might sometime make the coffee herself?

Mae: Well, sure.

Satir: Do you have to wait till she has to?

Mae: No, no. I don't think so.

Helen: I make the coffee at her house. She just . . .

Satir: What are you feeling right now, Mae?

Mae: I'm . . . I'm happy.

Satir: Uh-huh?

(Someone in background made sound with his tongue.)

Satir: Well, we have another little dialogue going on over here because . . . *(laughter)* . . . we are having something . . . it's all right, it's all right here . . . and what are you making?

Bill: Darrell?

Satir: It looks to me like you're making a doll of some sort. *(Darrell has been drawing.)*

Darrell: I am.

Satir: I thought you probably were. It looks like a pretty solid one. I'm wondering something. What are you feeling about what's going on here between your grandfather and your grandmother and your mother?

Darrell: I don't know.

Satir: What does it seem like to you? If you were to go to school tomorrow and tell people what went on here, what would you say what's going on here?

Darrell: *(long silence)* I don't know.

Satir: Your mother's been talking about growing up. Did you hear that?

Darrell: Uh-huh.

Satir: And your mother is . . . uh, has been talking to her father, your grandfather, and was talking something about how . . . she was glad to be growing up, and then she thought at some point that maybe, uh, she didn't grow up as fast as she might because your grandfather, her father, didn't always give her the opportunity. Did you hear that? Yeah. Did you notice how your grandfather responded when she said that? He was surprised! Because he didn't have any idea he was stopping her from growing up or . . . making her think he was stopping her. Did you notice that? Well, I did. Did you notice that, Maria? You noticed that. I think you'd like to come up here and be into this a little bit more. So maybe if you'd come a little closer to me, Darrell, right here . . . just scoot over a little bit . . . that's right.

Mae: *(Maria says something very softly—I can't understand it.)* It's hard having two grandchildren, one Darrell and one Maria.

Satir: Y-y-es. So how is that for you now, Maria? Coming up here and being a part of all this? (long silence) Where are you right now, Helen?

Helen: Worried about Darrell.

Satir: What are you worried about?

Helen: Un . . . I'm wondering if he doesn't know what he's feeling or if he . . . doesn't want to say what he's feeling.

Satir: Should I share with you my perception of what's going on here?

Helen: Um hum.

Satir: You worried a long time about whether you could grow up and maybe you could talk to your father the way you wanted to.

Helen: Um hum.

Satir: And I wonder how you feel about how available he is to you. You had some ideas that you thought he had, that it turned out he didn't have. Is that true or not true?

Helen: Yes. That's true.

Satir: Now what I hear you doing, I hear you doing something similar with Darrell. Do you know what I'm talking about?

Helen: Not letting it be.

Satir: That's one of the things. I think you're expecting Darrell to share something with you, and I'd be interested if you'd tell me, because this really has a lot to do with Darrell . . .

Helen: Um hum.

Satir: . . . what do you think he's supposed to tell you about how he feels? What are you waiting for?

Helen: Good question. *(long silence)*

Satir: What do you think he's holding back from you?

Helen: Anger.

Satir: Anger. He's angry with you? All right. Now, let's go into a little thing . . . with this. If you were in Darrell's shoes, why would you be angry with you?

Helen: What I worry about him being angry about . . . ?

Satir: Um hum . . .

Helen:. . . is . . . thinking that I . . . did something to make his Dad leave.

Satir: So you think that Darrell thinks that you did something to make his father go.

Helen: That's my fear.

Satir: All right. What do you think that he thinks you did? Might be true, but I don't know about it yet. What do you think that he thinks you did?

Helen: *(long silence)* Didn't love him . . . is the first thing that comes to my mouth.

Satir: You think that Darrell thinks: If my mother loved my father, my father wouldn't have gone. Is it something like that?

Helen: Yeah. That doesn't ring true, though, when I hear you say it.

Satir: OK. I just gave you back your words.

Helen: Yeah. My . . . gut reaction to that is oh, whew, let's start that all over.

Satir: What are you feeling now about where Darrell is?

Helen: I'm translating a feeling that I had about my dad . . . to Darrell at this moment, and that is, and this fits in with what Susan Arnold said about quitting taking care of Daddy. And I'm feeling the sense of relief I had yesterday when he came into this group and functioned just fine and I didn't have to make a bridge for him, which I felt I would have to do and have done in.

Satir: Susan just appeared in the interview. Should we bring her on the stage? Susan Arnold?

Helen: It's not real important to me.

Satir: OK. So something that you got through Susan is now something of yours?

Helen: Yes.

Satir: So let's deal with it that way. If you don't mind.

Helen: OK.

Satir: Are you aware that I'm also giving you some signals that you can take things on your own . . . a little bit more of what you were telling your father, that you could stand on your own feet?

Helen: That . . . I don't need Susan?

Satir: Well, you might need her, but right now what you're doing is to get whatever you took from her and using it for yourself.

Helen: Yes. Yes, I am. And the sense of relief that I had yesterday, and a deep relaxation in me that I haven't had . . . when we've been sharing any activities that wasn't work around the house or play in the sense of playing games with the kids, and that was just being, that, my gosh it's OK.

Satir: I'd like you to look at Darrell and give him, in your mind, the same freedom. And what does that feel like to you?

Helen: *(long silence)* It feels like a surrender.

Satir: Surrender? I don't know what that means.

Helen: It feels like a letting go of my stomach muscles that, um, he too can function on his own and respond however he damn well pleases. And, uh, for me that means that it's OK in a way to be alone and who I am, because the other way is when he's an extension of me, and I'm wanting to show off the parts of him that I want to be seen.

Satir: All right. Now this minute, Russell is sitting over there. Now, don't look, I want you to stay here. Russell is sitting over there. He's someone outside of this family, right?

Helen: Um hum.

Satir: Now, what are the chances for Darrell and Maria to have time, experience, and relationship with Russell as it is now worked out?

Helen: . . . on this stage . . .

Satir: In our life. What are the chances for those kids?

Helen: The chances are . . .

Satir: What are they now able to do?

Helen: They're able to see him sporadically if he comes into town, and they're able to call him if they want to or talk . . . although . . . *(Someone whispers: Mommy. What? Darrell . . . does it hurt? Just for a little bit more, honey. No.)*

Satir: Wait a minute now. Maria is at this point making some kind of request. Let's take a minute to look at what that request means. What do you think that she is asking you Helen?

Helen: I think she's asking me to quit talking about Russell. That it's more . . .

Satir: Well, what was she literally saying?

Helen: Take off the microphone.

Satir: Oh, OK. All right. We can look for the interpretations later.

Helen: *(laughs)* OK.

Satir: She's saying take off the microphone. Are you willing to do that?

Helen: Sort of.

Satir: Not really?

Helen: Not really.

Satir: But you took it off.

Helen: That's 'cause I was wanting to please you. But I'd like to talk to Maria about it, for a minute.

Satir: Go right ahead.

Helen: Maria, honey, can you put this on so if you talk we can hear? You don't want to do that? OK.

Satir: So where is that now with you?

Helen: I'm not going to ram the microphone on my daughter.

Satir: Now you had another thought, that something was going on in Maria's mind . . .

Helen: Um hmm.

Satir: . . . as you were talking about Russell. Can you give me your fantasy about what that was.

Helen: Uh-huh. That it was . . . um . . . my fantasy is that it's uncomfortable for her . . . and she doesn't like to hear it. Especially if it's real present tense, if we talk in terms of things we used to do, or, "Oh, your dad likes tennis or he likes this," then that's OK.

Satir: Now I have this feeling, and I want to share it with you. I don't know if it fits or not, but that this separation has only taken place as fact, that it hasn't really taken place in terms of all that it means, and I have this strong feeling I'm sure that Maria and Darrell have some questions and so on because I have the feeling that these are . . . you're talking about the children, but you're meaning yourself. Does that have any value or validity?

Helen: Yes.

Satir: All right. Let's try something. What's that click about?

Helen: That's Maria. Honey . . .

Satir: Oh.

Helen: Honey, don't . . .

Satir: Oh. OK.

Helen: . . . Don't . . . just put it down . . .

Satir: . . . So if you don't wear it, if you don't wear it, then you have to put it down. You can give it to the man over there or you can have it available to yourself when you want it again. I'd like you to turn your chair around and look at Russell.

Helen: Y . . . y . . . ea . . . h.

Helen: Yeah.

Satir: Well, he's right behind you so you can ask him . . . how he feels *(microphone shrieks. Someone goes, "aaaa")*

Helen: How do you feel about the anger, I'd . . . wait a minute . . . . I'm gonna turn back around to Grandpa . . .

Bill: Well, do you want me to answer that question?

Helen: Yeah.

Bill: I thought it was good.

Satir: Well, now, we're into an interesting thing here . . .
(laughter)

Helen: Maria, would you like to stand up?

Satir: Would you like to see your father's face?

Helen: Yes, I would.

Satir: OK.

Bill: I thought it was good.

Helen: Did you disagree with any of that?

Bill: No. I didn't disagree.

Helen: I mean, do you disagree with what I said when I said those, the angry things to Russell?

Bill: Yes, I think you're right.

Satir: Do you have anything to add of your own?

Bill: Well, I'd liked to have shot him. Where is he? Then I let my conscience at least take over. *(laughter)*

Satir: Why are you angry? From your place? Can you tell Russell why you're angry? At least, that part *(microphone shrieks)* . . . angry. *(Satir invites Bill to look at and directly face Russell.)*

Bill: Well, because my daughter gave up so much to help you get the position you hold today. She gave up an awful lot. I gave up an awful lot. My wife gave up an awful lot. When you needed help, we were always there, even more so than your own mother and dad. I remember when they first moved up to Peoria, they called . . .

Satir: Hey. When you first moved . . .

Bill: When you first moved up to Peoria, you asked me to help you unload the truck, the moving van there, and I never carried so many books in my life, from that truck over to the elevator, and then up the elevator and into the apartment. But I did all these things for love, well if you loved my daughter, this is why I was so angry when you went and threw all this away. Not only did you hurt us, you hurt your own parents.

Satir: How do you feel about what your father is saying right now?

Helen: *(long silence)* . . . I feel that the anger is real broad and real true. I guess that the thing, the finishing sentence that I kept hearing, kept waiting for is, "And, darn it, Russell after you left we wrote you three letters saying "if this is God's will, we understand that and we love you, and we always loved you as a son," and he has never ever spoken a word to them. Or acknowledged them in any way their existence.

Satir: OK. What were you feeling as you heard your father express his anger to Russell?

Helen: Um. I don't feel . . . that I gave up as much as you feel I gave up.

Bill: *(laughs)* Well, uh . . .

Helen: Which doesn't mean that I don't feel the anger, but that I just don't feel that, because, because of what I gained through my marriage.

Bill: Well . . . those were just some of the things that , uh, popped in my mind.

Helen: I think they're valid and true, and I felt good to hear you saying it.

Satir: What are you feeling right now towards your dad?

Helen: Kinda . . . relief . . . I don't know . . . relief. You know, I'm thinking about this fantasy. What I'm thinking about was during the ice storm, because this all happened during the ice storm. *(laughs)* And, uh, luckily he brought down an R2D2 punching bag and we beat the crap out of it. And I'm remembering that. I'm having that feeling. It was such a funny wordless thing that we all did it and it was just . . . the right thing at that time.

Satir: What are you aware of feeling right now, Mae?

Mae: Ahhh. Well, I want to talk to . . . *(whispering, then laughter)* Someone says "I'm going to move out of the way."
(more laughter)

Mae: *(Talking to Russell)* The first time we went down, Bill and I, after you left her, we had quite a time with the ice storm. She had no lights, she had nothing, no heat. But you, Russell, were in a warm apartment, and you didn't even come to take the children, to take care of them so they could be warm. Until some friend of Helen's told him, and he knew it, that you'd better get those children so they won't catch cold. And then another time we came down and I wrote you a letter—and I've written many mean ones since in my mind—but this was a nice one, saying that we missed you at the dinner table, and when we came down, and that we would always love you. And I heard nothing from you, not a thing, and haven't, for 2 ½ years. I haven't heard from you. And I loved you . . . as a son. And I felt we should have had some consideration. From you.

Satir: *(to role-playing Russell.)* I'm wondering if you can say something about your feelings as you hear your former father-in-law and mother-in-law, who were like parents in some respects, and your wife talk at this point. I wonder if you have anything that you could share in the way of your feelings.

Russell: I'll have to respond as I was responding to each of the different messages. To Helen's responses, I really didn't quite understand what she was saying. Part of me was passive and easy and part of me was aggressive and egotistical and I should have done this and I should have done that, and I didn't care and through the whole thing, through part of this whole thing, I felt like I was under some sort of conspiracy. *(child whispering)*

Satir: Hold it just one minute because you're not being heard because something is happening here with Maria and with Helen *(child whispers).* Is there something that you're hearing from Maria . . .

Helen: She wants me to come with her, and I'm wondering if that means going to the bathroom. . .

Satir: Well, you can ask her a direct question.

Helen: Uh-huh. Do you have to go to the bathroom, honey? Are you just tired and want to walk for a minute? Do you want to go for a walk with Martha, the woman that gave you your nametag? Would you like to go make a new nametag with Martha for a minute? And then come back? Do you see her? She's coming? . . . Go for a walk with Martha and go get your orange and have a little bit of pop that's over on the table? Go over with Martha for a minute, and you can come back whenever you want to.

Bill: Don't touch the microphone.

Satir: What was that like for you, for you to be aware that something else was going on and you had half attention over there and half attention on her? What was that like for you now that you look back on it?

Helen: Familiar.

Satir: And it's familiar, something you knew before. And what is the experience? Of trying to be in two places at once?

Helen: I tune out. From all of it.

Satir: How did you feel about the fact that I stopped, so that you could hear more of what was going on?

Helen: I felt like, I felt relieved and I also felt like, "Oh, Helen don't you know that if you're going toward wholeness as a person you would have done that for yourself? You blew it. On the going towards wholeness."

Satir: You're doing what you ought to do or whether you're not. OK. So you just blew it for yourself?

Helen: That was a quickie flash, but yes.

Satir: All right. Well, let's make a little check on that, and then turn our backs on it, OK?

Helen: Uh-huh.

Satir: We can get rid of it that way.

Helen: That's fine with me.

Satir: Now, as you look back on the experience of feeling, of now knowing that maybe you could have done something for yourself at that time, but you didn't . . .

Helen: Uh-huh.

Satir: How was it that it got accomplished anyway?

Helen: You intervened and than I felt free to, uh, interact with her and come to a decision that would satisfy what was needed.

Satir: And how does that feel for you right now?

Helen: Good!

Satir: OK. Cause the first time I asked you, you got yourself into a self-blame thing.

Helen: Um hum.

Satir: And that's neither good nor bad. I just would like to have you know more clearly where you are in a moment in time. Somewhere along the line, you got the idea that you ought to do all things for all people and all the time, I gather.

Helen: Uh-huh.

Satir: Now the second time I asked you, when you clarified some things, you could feel that you had an experience from which you can grow. The scoreboard doesn't really matter, does it?

Satir: Do it from here.

Satir: Now when you look at this distance to Russell right now, just what are you aware of, Helen?

Helen: *(long silence)* Sadness.

Satir: Sadness. OK.

(Someone whispers, "that's OK".)

Satir: Could you put any words to that sadness, dear?

(Whispering.)

Helen: I feel . . . sad . . . oh . . . for the beauty that was, and, uh, my responsibility in it . . .

Satir: What was that?

Helen: What?

Satir: What was that responsibility?

Helen: I feel a lack of consciousness, an unawareness of what . . . . I've taken for granted . . . a lack of consciousness of the preciousness . . .

Satir: Are you having regrets?

Helen: Uh . . .

Satir: Could you share those regrets and whatever *(microphone shrieks)* Yeah. Yeah. When you get close up there it makes those sounds, so maybe you lean your head on that shoulder. Could you put into words those regrets?

Helen: *(long silence)* I regret, um, not having seen him more clearly. I regret . . . not having loved you well enough. *(turning to role-playing Russell)*

Satir: Do you really think he went away because he was unloved and unseen? Is that where you are with that?

Helen: *(long silence)* . . . I'm having a big fight in the head at this point . . .

Satir: All right. Close your eyes, look at the fight and tell me what's going on.

Helen: . . . one side's saying, "You jerky lady, you're berserk, he was having an affair with your best friend. Are you nuts? That's why he went away. Why are you taking all this on yourself. Um . . . also, he's a very egotistical and genuinely selfish guy, and he just kinda didn't like the whole family thing, and yes, he loves the kids, when they're right in front of him, but the rest of the time ignores them." And the other side is saying, "I don't care about those factors, I care about my part, and the things that I did and the consciousness I now have of what loving means versus what I had . . . when

I took the relationship for granted." *(microphone shrieks)* . . . I have *(Helen closes eyes.)*

Satir: All right. Now close your eyes again and watch it and see if any progress gets made and who wins, which side?

All right. Now, 'cuz I see it so strong the side's winning that's saying, "Cut the crap, Helen what *(laughs)* . . . uh . . ."

All right. Be with that for a moment. How do you feel about letting yourself know about the negative parts of your experience?

Helen: Angry!

Satir: All right. So look at him now, and give words to that anger. *(Helen turns to Russell)*

Helen: I'm angry that you were so incredibly passive, and that you took the preciousness of the three of us and never dealt with it directly at all and flipped off sideways, and, uh, in a way that was humiliating to me, and incredibly . . . brusque, and selfish and obnoxious . . . and I'm angry that you so totally discounted me . . .

Satir: What are you feeling in here now? As you're getting . . .

Helen: More anger. And more relief.

Satir: OK. What other kinds of angers come forward?

Helen: And I'm angry, that, um, for all the times that I . . . in a way I didn't perceive you right, I kept coming with a sort of problem-solving. The family is a wonderful place to learn and love and grow and offering that to you, and let's talk in this area of growth, and how can we do it, and how can we grow, and inside you were really sitting there and saying, I want to go play tennis, I want to go find some lady . . . and, um, and I'm angry at myself that I didn't perceive that and I kept pouring all this down the disposal.

Satir: How do you feel now that he's in his context and you're in your own?

Helen: More angry, more able to be angry.

Satir: Now how do you think your father feels about your anger toward Russell?

Helen: I think he'd like to put up big flags and go *(imitates the sound of a bugle).* Go get it, say it some more jump, biff, bam, boom.

Satir: He'd be on your side?

Helen: Yes.

Satir: . . . telling him what an awful guy he is?

Helen: No.

Satir: How does that feel for you?

Helen: A big relief. Like free fall. Different. A really different space that I've ever existed in.

Satir: OK. I'd just like you now, just let yourself relax, and I'd like you now to hear what our role-playing Russell has to say.

Russell: Do I begin again, or continue where I left off?

Helen: Just a minute. You can sit on the floor too, if you want to.

Russell: With Helen, I wasn't really clear of the messages that you were giving me. I felt like I was one person at one time, I was a different person at another time, and that I never ever had any feelings about anything, and when I listened to Darrell. . .

(Helen talks to child)

Satir: Bill or Mae?

Russell: Bill. It was like I was hearing a lot of love messages, but I wasn't really picking up love, you know, the tone of voice and the way you were handing it to me, it was just like I was, like I felt like I was, a misfit, like you did it for me in the name of something that I didn't really feel, like it was really together on it. Like I was still devoid of feelings, all I wanted was everything I could get from anybody, and that I never had any sense of appreciation and any sense of caring about anyone except myself. And, then, it just really made me feel low, and I just really felt bad about that, but I can't believe that it's true, because I do have feelings. And even though I may not have done all the right things, I still care about these kids. I was thinking, you know, how can anybody not love them? You were making me feel like I never had, and I never could. And, Mae, you just, when you talked, and already experienced all of this other stuff, by the time you told me about the letters, all I could feel was guilt. But I didn't have anything to respond with. 'Cause I really felt all of it was going on, you know, with the other person, and those were the messages that I was getting. That's the way I felt.

Satir: What are you feeling right now, inside?

Russell: I really feel nervous . . . kinda . . . like I'm all by myself.

Satir: I'd like to ask you, Bill, something. Is anything that this role-playing Russell is saying that you know about yourself in terms of feeling? Feeling outside and feeling not cared

about, having disappointed someone. Do you know anything about those kinds of feelings? Have you ever had any
experience in your life where you felt some of those feelings?

Mae: Are you asking him or me?

Satir: I'm asking Bill.

Bill: You mean like rejection, and . . .

Satir: Uh hum.

Bill: *(long silence)* Yeah, but right now I can't think of anything,
any one specifically.

Satir: But there's a familiarity on some level, I hear you saying.
And I wonder what you were feeling inside as you were
hearing Russell talk.

Bill: Well, I was wondering whether I, uh, made a misjudgment .
. . Some of the things that he did say *(whispering between
Helen and child)* . . . maybe I somehow wave-lengthed
those feelings, which, at the time I thought it was, we say,
because we love. *(more whispering)* And I'm a person that
likes to help people, and I expect nothing in return. But if I
can get a little love from it, that's the big payoff.

Satir: You know what I'm aware of, Bill, is the deep feeling of disappointment that you have in Russell.

Bill: Oh, well, I have.

Satir: I wonder if you could just share that with him, the real
deep feeling of disappointment.

Bill: Yes, I have a real down deep disappointment that . . . you
did these things. And as I said previously, that my Christian upbringing has taught me that you cannot bear hate,
you have to give love, or you will have a burning ulcer that
can make you ill.

Satir: I heard something else from you, Bill. I heard you say
something to the effect that you didn't have a son, and
that it looked like he might be the one. You might not have
said that directly, but I wonder if that wasn't what you
were feeling about Russell?

Bill: That I didn't have a son? Well, I thought I did at first. Especially while they, uh, went down to Haiti while they were
teaching in the Peace Corps. They, uh, had mom and dad
come down. And *(laughs)* at that time, Russell had a beard.

Satir: Come closer, Russell.

Bill: A beard just like you're wearing, see, and Helen had said
something, "Hey don't blow your cool." Now, having a

beard didn't bother me one bit. But, when I first saw Russell, first thing, he expected me to probably blow. But I said, "Hey, man, you look great, you really look like, you know, that smiling picture of Jesus Christ?" I said, "That's what you look like." And he, he didn't know what to say. He was taken back by that. He was a loveable guy.

Satir: Say "you" to him.

Bill: Huh?

Satir: Say "you" to him.

Bill: You were a lovable guy. We had a great time. I think you treated mom and dad like we were a couple of teenagers because we, ah, flew over to St. Thomas and there was no hotel, and we all said, well, we'll just sleep out on the beach. And, um, it seems after you got back and got through law school and started moving up the ladder, why, he started to be a changed person. And, uh, why we did those things, I don't know. Maybe this meeting here today might bring some of those things out. But, uh, we've avoided talking about . . . but . . . I really never got a chance to talk to you. You were gone. When it happened, I mean. We're maybe finding out a few things right here at this moment. That, uh, Helen has brought out. But in the meantime, I have . . . forgiven you. And even if—I've said this to Mae—that even if you were to come back, I'd love you again. Because I think you do have worth.

Satir: What do you feel about what you're hearing from Bill right now, Russell?

Russell: I heard you saying that you can forgive me, and that you could love me again, but I'm really concerned of just how much and what I would have to do in order to get that forgiveness and that love again.

Bill: Just come back.

Russell: Well, I don't know. I've just got a feeling that I've got an awful lot to do before I can ever fit back in again.

Bill: Well, love's not like that. I think you've all heard in First Corinthians, 13: "Love isn't a clanging cymbal." It's forgetting, and I've tried to live up to that. I've had lots of problems with it.

Russell: Bill, a few short moments ago, I had a lot of anger, and a lot of guilt imposed upon me. And now I'm hearing that it can all just happen like that, and I can't trust that right now. I just don't think you can forgive me that fast.

Bill: Well, you'll have to try. You'll have to try me. You see, that's
what I mean.

The interview continued. Bill was able to express both his
yearning to be loved by Russell and his anger toward him for not
allowing this to happen. This led into his anger toward his wife,
which, in turn, revealed the alliance between father and daughter.

The emphasis shifted to the pain in the relationship between
Bill and Mae, which made it possible for Helen to see how she felt
caught between her parents. Frank sharing of the pain and anger
in all three persons followed this. The children moved off quietly
and happily as their mother and grandparents took care of some
old business that served to keep Helen in a dependent role, which
she had duplicated in her relationship to her husband, Russell,
and now with her children. The depression seemed related to her
giving herself blame messages, apparently to protect her from the
anger and frustration she felt toward both of her parents, as well
as the unexpressed longing she had to be close to them. All of this
she had projected on her children.

In the interview, it becomes clear that Helen had not yet
transformed her ties to her family of origin. My effort was to re-
shape these ties so Helen could be more freely in charge of herself and her family and have more of a peer relationship with her
parents. In following up this case, I found that this indeed did
happen.

Helen was able to develop her own independent living arrangements with her children. Russell, her ex-husband, began
participating in the parenting of the children. Helen became
more of a peer with her parents, thus creating a more human
and mature relationship with them. Her depression lifted completely as she took charge of herself.

Evaluation

By now, I have seen close to 5,000 families of nearly every
shape, form, nationality, race, income group, religious orientation
and political persuasion.

I personally have done no formal research on my results. I
have left that to others. What I know about the effectiveness of
my work has come from my students and feedback from the
families that I have seen, which comes frequently and over time.
My feedback indicated that the results have been generally use-

ful, and seem to get more so. That is not to say that I have not fallen on my face. I have. But when I fail—and get over the pain of it - I find new learning for myself in the experience. I imagine that is how it will continue to be.

Summary

There always seems to be a keen interest in how therapists come to be what they are. In this chapter, I see myself as an avid observer and lover of people. I regard people as miracles and the life within them as sacred. I present a more or less chronological account of how I see myself becoming a family therapist. Of course, I realize that no one part of what I have presented is pivotal. Each part interacts with others and unites to form the possibility for seeing further.

In sharing with readers my search to know myself, to understand my family, and to help others, I share my awareness of how the strands of my life are reflected in my theoretical underpinnings and translated into my therapeutic approach and style. To convey my ideas about family therapy, I have chosen to write this chapter essentially as a chronicle of my journey of seeing and relating to people in need. Initially trained as a teacher and then as a psychiatric social worker, I am one of the unorthodox people who stumbled onto the possibility of working with the family as a treatment unit.

The outcome of my ongoing learning, at this point in time, is a process of family therapy in which the therapist and the family join forces to promote wellness among the family members. I call it the Process Model. The heart of the Process Model consists of all those interactions and transactions translated into methods and procedures that move the individuals in the family, and the family system itself, from a symptomatic base to wellness.

My basic assumption in the Process Method is that people are geared toward growth. A symptom, then, is an indication that the freedom to grow is being blocked by the rules in the family system and, in turn, limits the creative use of the context. The rules that govern the family system are derived from the ways in which parents maintain their self-esteem. These rules, in turn, form the context within which the children grow and develop their self-esteem. In my view, communication and self-worth are the base of the family system.

Since all systems are balanced, the question is: What price does each part of the system pay to keep it so? Any symptom, therefore, signals a blockage in growth and is connected to the survival of the system. The form of this survival connection differs with each individual and with each family, but the essence is the same. An early step in intervention is to make this system pattern visible, felt and understood.

My second assumption is that all human beings have within them all of the resources they need to flourish. My therapeutic process is to aid people in gaining access to their nourishing potentials and in learning how to use them. The use of these potentials is what creates a growth-producing system. To tap the potentials, I use eight levels of access: (1) physical, (2) intellectual, (3) emotional, (4) sensual, (5) interactional, (6) contextual, (7) nutritional, (8) spiritual.

The symptom gives me a starting point; it gives me clues for unraveling the net of distorted, ignored, denied, projected, unnourished, and untapped parts of each person so that they can connect with their ability to cope functionally, healthily and joyously.

A third assumption is that everyone and everything is impacted by—and impacts—everyone and everything in the system. I have developed methods to include all the people in a therapy session—in spirit, if not in body—who impact one another. There are multiple stimuli and multiple effects; therefore, there can be no blame. This is a fundamental human systems concept.

I act upon a fourth assumption, namely that (1) therapy is a process that takes place between persons in a positive and health-promoting context to accomplish a positive change and (2) the therapist can be expected to be the leader in initiating and teaching the health-promoting process in the family, but cannot take charge of the persons involved. The love and trust context that I develop with the family is the means by which I help people take the necessary risks to start taking charge of themselves. The process is weighted heavily toward each member of the family becoming as whole as possible.

To illustrate the Process Model, I included an excerpt from an initial interview with a family to show the ways in which I use my assumptions that people are indeed basic miracles and capable of change.

Annotated Selected Readings

I regard books as inspiration toward new possibilities, spring-boards to trying out new ideas, validation of one's own perceptions, further resources to add to one's current information reservoir and, many times, as guides for direction when one sees where one wants to go, and doesn't quite see how to get there. The following are a small selection which fulfill these functions. In turn, they can lead to further reading.

Bandler, R., Grinder, J., & Satir, V. (1976). *Changing with families*. Palo Alto, California: Science and Behavior Books.
Family therapy utilizing a neuro-linguistic approach.

Dodson, L. S. (1977). *Family counseling: A systems approach*. Muncie, Indiana: Accelerated Development.
A description of family process and dynamics from a Jungian base.

Luthman, S., & Kirschenbaum, M. (1974). *The dynamic family*. Palo Alto, California: Science and Behavior Books.
A beautiful, vital, and detailed presentation of family process in action.

Satir, V. (1967). *Conjoint family therapy* (Rev. ed.). Palo Alto, California: Science and Behavior Books.
A base within which to look at many aspects of the human "onion".

Satir, V. (1972). *Peoplemaking*. Palo Alto, California: Science and Behavior Books.
An account of universal factors in families, simply written to increase appreciation of what families are all about.

Satir, V., Stachowiak, J., & Taschman, H. (1977). *Helping families to change*. New York: Aronson.
A very specific and detailed account of treatment intervention.

Satir, V. *Self esteem*. (1975). Millbrae, California: Celestial Arts.

Satir, V. *Making contact*. (1976) Millbrae, California: Celestial Arts.

Satir, V. *Your many faces.* (1978) Millbrae, California: Celestial Arts.

All three of the above are written in a readable conversational manner aimed at helping the reader to become more richly aware of his or her humanness.

I urge the reader to also become acquainted with the writings of Nathan Ackerman, Jay Haley, Salvador Minuchin, Murray Bowen, and Don Jackson. They are readily available under the authors' names. I especially call attention to the book by Carl Whitaker and Gus Napier:

Napier, A.Y., Whitaker, C.A. (1978). The family crucible. Mew York: Harper and Row, Publishers, Inc.
This is a human and well written presentation of live experiences as family therapists.

There are three other books which I regard as very useful adjuncts to a therapist's education.

Gately, R., & Koulach, D. (1979). *The single father's handbook.* New York: Anchor Press/Doubleday.
In a readable, human way and practical manner these authors offer some important insights and some much needed perspective on single-parent families.

Rainwater, J. (1979) *You're in charge.* California: Guild of Tutors Press.
This author is a creative transactional analyst. In a light, practical and human way she draws attention to how parents can develop and use their power in a loving and effective way.

Visher, E., & Visher, J., (1979). *Stepfamilies.* New York: Brunner/Mazel.
This book is an attempt to establish legitimacy for the step-family. Given the number of children in our society who will be brought up in step-families the authors take a significant first step in making this an attractive and loving family form.

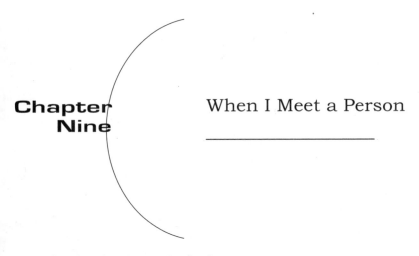

Chapter Nine

When I Meet a Person

Introduction by Jesse Carlock

Virginia Satir has been recognized as a master therapist and teacher, not only in the United States and Canada, but throughout the world. The article is, in my opinion, one of her best in that it distills the essence of her views on her transformational approach to therapy. I have studied her work for nearly 30 years and, of all her writings, I believe this is one that will truly whet your appetite for learning more about Satir and her ground-breaking approach to therapy and personal growth.

"When I Meet a Person" originally appeared in the book, _Tidings of Comfort and Joy_, edited by Robert Spitzer in 1975. In it, Satir paints a narrative picture of her work with a family, while it is still fresh in her mind. She describes her internal process from this, her first meeting with the family, as well as the ingredients she sees as vital in the change process. In the article, Satir is at her best. She reflects, in· an extemporaneous fashion, on her experience with this family, weaving together an interplay between her basic beliefs about people, her astute observations of behavior, and her images of what lies beneath the outer layers. She emphasizes reliance on her images, thoughts, feelings and sensations in the moment, and her sense about the energy field between and among all concerned.

To Satir, treatment sessions were a dynamic dialogue, lively experiences of human contact wherein the full person of the therapist meets the full person of the client. Each session was a novel *dance that, at its best, activated in clients an expanded vision of self and an ability to use self fully and connect with others in more meaningful ways. To Satir, no session was complete until some kind of transformation occurred or a new window opened for the client. She sought not only to change thoughts, feelings, and behavior, but more importantly, she reached for changes in the client's fundamental relationship with self.*

Satir firmly believed that without self-worth, change could not happen. Ahead of her time, and subject to much criticism for some of her beliefs, she was perhaps the first psychotherapist to address the spiritual dimension as part of the therapy process. Yet Satir maintained an unshakable belief that, regardless of whatever problems are manifest, every person has an unblemished core or life force. Her work consistently demonstrated that, when this life force is contacted, nurtured and developed in a context of caring and acceptance, people can flower. This repetitive theme of connecting with the self-worth of clients and reaching into their yearnings and longings appears again and again as a central theme in Satir's work. She shows in this article how she is able to see beyond the outside layers and tap the often hidden core life force in order to gauge her moves and activate change.

This central focus on contacting the life force, combined with her sharply honed self-awareness and data gathering ability using all sensory channels, represents the epitome in the use of all resources—self, other and the higher self—as dynamic instruments of change. Satir worked to achieve an enlightenment in every session. I am certain that this article will open doors for you as well.

■ ■ ■

People have often asked me how I look at people and what I see when I look. Many times what I think people are really asking is what kind of beliefs I have about people. I will try to answer this in a way that I think might help people understand more about some of the things that I do when I'm working with people. I will treat this in an extemporaneous fashion, trying to put together what I do as thoughts occur to me. I am quite aware that many of the ways I feel and the things I do may not be all that's there, but I will share with you the best that I know at this point.

I would like to start with what goes on in me when I think about using myself as a helper to another person. In the first place, the person and his family—because I almost always think in the family context—would not be coming to me unless they had some kind of pain or some kind of problem that they wanted to solve. In some way I feel them as having said to themselves (or having been told by someone else), "We've reached the end of our ability to cope, and we are searching for some way to cope better." People don't always put it in that language. Sometimes they only say, "I hurt" or "Somebody is doing something wrong." I hear it as a search for a new ability to cope better with their lives, and to have more joy and pleasure, less pain, and perhaps more productivity.

I see all people as representations of life, in whatever form that happens to be. When people are in need or are having some kind of problem, their manifestation of themselves—the way they look and sound and talk—can be pretty ugly, pretty beautiful, or pretty painful. Underneath all this I see the living human who, I feel, would use himself or herself differently if he or she were in touch with the life that he or she is and has. So with every human being that I encounter, I mentally take off his or her outside and try to see the inside, which is that piece of the self that I call self-worth or self-esteem, and to which I have given the affectionate name *pot*. This pot is searching for some way of manifesting itself, and I meet a person with that awareness. There is in the person that which probably he or she has not touched. That person not only hasn't touched it, he or she doesn't even know it's there. I know it's there. This conviction in me is so strong that it is a given for me. I never ask if that person has life; I ask only how it can be touched.

Yesterday I did an interview with a family that is fresh in my mind at the moment. What I am going to try to do is describe, in the best way I can, what happened between the family and me. I'll supply my understanding of what was going on in me, and how I used that understanding to reach the self-worth of each member of the family. This family had an adult male and an adult female, who were husband and wife. These two adults were also the father and mother of five children, the oldest eighteen and the youngest five. Of course, they had some kind of problem or they wouldn't have come in for treatment. That part was also obvious.

To start off, I was not so much concerned with a particular problem as with trying to understand and learn about how each person in this family lived his or her life, both with the others and with him or herself. For me, there are always two lives going on all the time—mine with myself, and mine with the other people who are significant to me. When I met this family, I didn't know what I was going to find. I did not know how these particular family members were going to manifest themselves; I only knew that they were hurting and that they had something in them that could be touched and developed and that could grow.

The first thing I did was to meet each one. Something that I am quite aware of is that people aren't usually related to themselves as people of worth. I feel that no changes can be made in people unless they begin to feel themselves as having worth, and that I, as the therapist, become the first means by which a person comes in touch with his or her own feeling of worth. My meeting with this family was the beginning of this. I extended my hand to the husband-father, and subsequently did the same with all the rest of the family.

I would like to say a little bit about what it was like for me when I did that. In the first place—and you might think along with me—suppose you are someone I am just meeting. You are with a group of people, perhaps members of your family, and I stand in front of you and reach out my hand to you at arm level. As I reach for your hand and you give it to me, I feel a connection. At that moment in time, I am looking at you; I am in touch with your skin feelings and my skin feelings and, for that moment, there is no one else in the world except you and me. You are the receiver of my full attention at that moment. You can feel that what I am connecting with is your personhood, and I feel that I am giving mine to you. A smile accompanies this, and my smile is saying "hello" to you and to your life as a representation of all life. This kind of experience makes it possible for me to feel that I am connected with another form of life—another manifestation of life—yours. I regard life manifestation as the basis of what personhood is all about.

As I do this with each member of your family, I am also aware, within myself, that I am enjoying having the contact—full contact—which in some way also affirms me. I am a living being connected with another living being. It is like the platform, or the base, from which we are going to go. This is why I do not start out my treatment session with a discussion of the problem, but rather make this basic connection on a human level with everyone. Of course, people are coming in for some help; if they knew what sort of help they needed, they would probably be doing it themselves and not seeking me. They have come to the end of their coping and they want some help, but probably all that they are aware of is that they have pain.

As I am making this first contact with them, I am listening to their responses to me. In a few moments, I will hear responses from the people to each another. I begin to get a feeling for what they have done, for how they have used their experiences from the time they popped out of the womb until now. Some of you may be familiar with the *stances* I use for shorthand purposes, the ways in which people communicate with one another. These responses I have labeled as *placating, blaming, super-reasonable, irrelevant,* and *flow*. At the beginning of treatment I do not expect the family to display many flow responses, because the fact that they haven't arrived at that point is probably one of the reasons they are coping in the way that they are. I also want to under-score the fact that I see the people in front of me as doing the very best they can with what they have learned; and I believe that what they have learned represents the best way they know how to survive. Some of you may be aware that I have translated the various kinds of responses into *body positions*. Within a few moments, I am making mental pictures of the people in front of me and translating them into physical postures that represent their ways of communicating.

For example, in the family I saw yesterday, I saw the man as making super-reasonable responses. That meant that, in my imagination, he was standing there very erect, with very little movement, speaking in a rather monotonous way. I saw the woman kneeling before him in a placating position, but at the same time, behind her back, pointing an accusing finger at him. I saw the oldest daughter standing and super-reasonable like her father, looking at neither parent but with one finger barely pok-ing out, pointing at her father. I saw the next girl very deliber-ately, and in a very obvious way, pointing her finger at her mother. The next child was a boy. I saw him standing very close to his mother and placating her. Then I saw the next child as giv-ing out irrelevant responses by moving all over the place and not being able to fix on anyone. I also saw the youngest child, a five-year-old girl, as being irrelevant.

As I saw these pictures in my mind, it was important to re-spect them as representing the best ways that these people had developed to cope. Their ways of placating, blaming, and being super-reasonable or irrelevant had formed a system that meant that no one in the family could really approach the personhood of another. They were likely to mishear one another; they were seeing roles rather than real people. So my search and any efforts would be directed to helping these people to become real with one another. I looked at this family, and my insides felt them respond to my contact. Full contact, by the way, carries the message of caring—caring in a deep, personal sense—and I regard that contact as a vital basis for developing any changes. There has to be high trust. If people in the family group do not find me trustworthy, I don't think we are going to be able to affect any changes.

I remember that, as I entered the room yesterday, the family was spread around on chairs, looking very much like targets on a rifle range. A table was in front of them. As I looked at this scene, I felt that it would be very awkward to work in this context. I feel very strongly that where people are sitting (far apart or close together) and the way they are sitting is very important. I need to make the place where I work comfortable, that is, to arrange it so that I can see everybody. I place myself within arm's length of each person. There must be enough space for me and the other people to move about. This space is necessary because sometimes I will have family members work in pairs, or I will do sculpturing or some other kind of activity that requires space. A table or other obstacle makes movement difficult. Yesterday, I moved the table and fixed it so that I was no more than a small step away from making touch contact with everyone in the group.

The little five-year-old was on my right. At one point I noticed that she was moving back a little bit. By this time I had the feeling that she was regarded as the troublemaker in the family and was rather on the outside. I slipped my hand around her back—she had a nice, round back—and I found myself feeling the enjoyment of touching her. I think she felt this as a message of encouragement to be a part of the group. Throughout the interview there was much more of this.

One can touch in all kinds of ways. In training therapists, I have told them that to develop "eyes and ears" in their fingers is important. People in families are touching all the time—slapping, pushing, shoving, holding. I'm sure all of you know that touches have different meanings. So it isn't a matter of giving a touch; it's a matter of the message in the touch.

I referred earlier to developing trust. That means that the atmosphere, through trust, has to be such that people can begin to talk about what I call unspeakable things; the things that are close to their hearts, what they worry about, what they fear, and what they hope for. I don't know if I can state this strongly enough. To me, that people do say what was once unspeakable is much more important than what they say. Sometimes it takes a little while for people to get the feeling that whatever they say can be heard and understood. It does not have to be run through any censorship system about what is right. I don't know of any way to help a person get to himself or herself unless that person can let out whatever is there. That is not a usual thing in this society, as many of you doubtlessly know. But to create the context and the working way for change to take place, it seems to me that no one can be penalized, in any way, for what he or she says—at least not by me. Instead, I must take whatever someone says and make a living account of where the person is at that moment. What that person says must be understood by him or her as well as by everyone else. This means that a great deal of clarifying must go on so that a family can understand what each member is really trying to say.

As yesterday's interview proceeded, I put a question to each person in the family: "What do you hope will happen to you as a result of your coming here?" I suppose the usual question a therapist might ask is, "What is the problem?" I am interested in finding out where people are locked in, but I also feel that my way of asking about this, and what I ask, helps the person to center more on himself or herself. It also goes a little way toward diminishing the negative "vibes" that are usually there—usually in some form of "Well, if he or she were better, I would be better," or something of that sort.

In this instance I started out with the oldest daughter. At this moment I don't know why I did, except that at the time it seemed to be the right place to start. She said that she would like to see the family "not fight so much." I went on to her sister, who said the same thing. I asked other family members if they had noticed that there was a lot of fighting going on. Everyone acknowledged this. The next picture that emerged in my mind was of the two older girls fighting with one another. It seemed, at that point, that they were the focus around which the family's problems centered. The argument was that if these two girls didn't fight, then the family would be better. What this introduced was how the people in this family would be comfortable about expressing their anger. When I put my question to the father, his answer was that his family needed to be educated on things they had previously not known.

Because I like to make an "alive" picture as quickly as possible, it seemed natural at that point to ask the two older girls to get up and point their fingers at each other in order to see what other family members did when this happened. I find that words are more useful when there is a picture; I call this *sculpturing* or *posturing*. I found that when I asked the two girls to point at each other, they were very reluctant to do so. They talked about how they fought, but actually putting themselves in the position of doing it made it more real. They seemed embarrassed.

One of the important things that I try to do is help people to be free (I am using "free" in the sense of having options and choices). I encourage people to start playing with new ideas about their behavior. I give them support to break through their taboos. Since the two girls were embarrassed, I stood behind the girl who seemed most embarrassed and supported her, standing close to her back and taking her arm and helping it to go out in a pointing direction. Then I did the same thing for the other girl. I was essentially taking the first step toward breaking this family's rule that you shouldn't be angry. This then led to the matter of what the others in the family do when there is fighting. Here were the two girls standing and pointing at each other, and everyone in the family had seen this before. My next question to the husband-father was, "What do you do when this happens?" He said he tried to tell the girls to stop, but it didn't do any good. I had him come up with his finger pointing and, when he saw that this did no good either, he dropped his and sat down. One of the girls said the wife-mother "came on a little stronger," so I had her come in with her finger pointing. I asked some of the other children what usually happened. They said they tried to stay out of it. The oldest boy now went to his mother's side, so he came in like an auxiliary father, trying to help her with the problem between the two girls.

This kind of sculpturing has value because it makes explicit what is going on. It also brings the present (but not acknowledged) family process picture to life. This picture is not to show how bad people are, but to help them see what is going on. There is oftentimes a good bit of humor in this. I remember at one point asking the oldest girl to put out her finger. Her hand was a little wobbly, so I supported it and asked her to make believe there really was a pistol at the end of her hand. Lighthearted things like this tend to help neutralize the negative self-worth effect and to increase the ability of the person to look and to see. For me, it is very important to make the separation between the person, his or her values, and how he or she is using himself or herself. I am bringing people in touch with the various ways they use themselves as well as with how they can use themselves differently. I do this in ways that raise their feelings of self-worth.

People often ask me if I feel drained after an interview. My answer is "No." I would get drained if I kept asking myself all kinds of questions like, "Am I doing it right? Will people love me? Am I going to come out with a cure?" If I started to do that (which I call potting myself), I would lose track of the system and process that are going on and I would be on my story rather than the story of the family.

This leads me now to something else. I consider myself the leader of the process in the interview but not the leader of the people. I check out everything I do with them before I do it. I am a strong leader for the process. This is based on the fact that I am the one who knows what the process I am trying to produce is all about. I want to help people to become their own designers of their own choice-making; before they can do that, they need to be free to take risks. My checking out with them their willingness to undertake something new is a very important piece of this interaction and alerts them to the experience of taking risks. If I have something to offer you, I need to tell you about it; I need to show you; I need to ask you if what I offer has any value to you. What is important is that if I am introducing something new to you and I ask you too soon if you are willing to do it—that is, before I have gotten your understanding, trust, and willingness to take risks - then you will not be in a place where you feel that you can take a chance.

People often say to me, "Well, what if something you do backfires?" I answer, "That's not unusual." It is what happens in life when you try something that doesn't work. You have some choices after that. You can call yourself bad names for trying it out, or you can use it as a life experience and learn from it. Nothing backfired in yesterday's interview because it seemed that I was in the flow and had nice things going. That is the whole point. As a therapist, I try to be aware of what is happening and keep it flowing rather than try continually to keep score of what is right or wrong.

This might be a good place to say that when I am speaking to a family, I am not trying to solve a specific problem, such as should they get a divorce or should they have a baby. I am working to help people find a different kind of coping process. I do not see myself as wise enough to know what is the best thing for a person to do. Should the wife ask her mother-in-law to leave? Should she demand that she leave? Should the wife leave her husband if the mother-in-law doesn't behave? These kinds of questions are not mine to answer. My task is to help each person with his or her own coping, so that he or she can decide to do the things that work for him or her.

In yesterday's family, it came out that the second girl occasionally talked of committing suicide. A lot of hate responses were going on between her and her mother. Instead of responding to that hate, I read in my insides that these two people wanted very much to get a connection with each other but there were all kinds of barriers between them. I had learned earlier that the wife-mother had viewed this particular child as having the same problems she had had, and was feeling very sad about seeing them in her child. Apparently the mother was trying to solve the problems in herself by trying to solve them in her daughter. This, of course, was why these two could not get together.

I asked the two of them to move toward each other, because by this time the trust level was sufficiently established so that they would be willing to take this risk. First I had them move to where they could see each other clearly, approximately at arm's length, and then I had them look at each other. I then had them close their eyes and I asked each of them to tell me what she saw. This was very interesting. The wife-mother said she saw a little baby whom she hadn't cared for very well, and that she was feeling very guilty. She began to sob a little. When I asked the daughter what she had seen, she said first that she just saw her mother. Then, after her mother had spoken, the girl said, "Well, she always sees me as a baby."

What I was aware of at this point was that these two were not seeing each other as they really were at this point in time; they were seeing each other in terms of past experience. If they didn't change, they would continue to see each other in this way and problems between them would escalate.

One of the criticisms that the daughter had made earlier was that her mother always treated her like a little baby. After this disclosure, I pointed out to the mother that she was indeed seeing this thirteen-year-old as a baby. Then, after asking the mother her age, I pointed out to the daughter that she was seeing a thirty-six-year-old person. I stated that there were these two ladies (I used that word), Cynthia and June, who were looking at each other. I wondered out loud if they would see each other as Cynthia and June. Then I asked them to look again and tell me, after shutting their eyes, what they saw.

They were being what I call brought up to date. As June (the mother) spoke, she said she saw this thirteen-year-old who was attractive and that it was a whole new awareness for her. The daughter said she saw her mother and the look in her eyes—which seemed to be a look of caring for her—and which she liked. Both of them at that point said they felt a whole lot different about one another.

The family then moved on to another situation involving the older daughter and her father. She was almost eighteen, and her father was still insisting that she come home early. It turned out that this man, because of his psychological and physical problems, had not yet come to a place where he could see himself as supporting his family by his work alone. His wife was working from 2:30 in the afternoon until midnight or so, which meant that the bulk of the management of the family was in the hands of the husband. He had worked out with the older daughter that she cooked dinner. Apparently she did the shopping, too. He demanded that she come home early, which she felt was an affront, kind of invasion.

I asked these two to sit in front of one another and just try to hear one another. I guided their listening and helped them to see that they were not talking to each other in terms of what the other was saying, but only in terms of how each wanted to control the other. After this, it seemed as though both the daughter and her father had come to a new understanding.

It was quite clear at this point that both the husband and wife were very fearful about what would happen to their children. Another piece of information that came out was that both of them had parents who had left them early. They were both brought up by grandparents who apparently were very anxious about them. This anxiety was transferred. Without this being clear before, most of the children in the family heard the parents' efforts to care for them as something against them. They had not been in touch with this other part. At the same time, the parents had been hearing their children as being quarrelsome and unappreciative. We were able to make some new connections.

Throughout the interview, my mental picture was one of content flowing out and connections being made. Using myself in a very active way, I could pick out times (as with the mother and daughter) to make a new connection. During the flow of touching in the family, the mother said that she hoped that her youngest son would hug her. When he came home, he only gave her a "little old hug" and she always felt cheated. The whole question of affection in the family and how people could be affectionate was brought up. This had had a taboo on it. At the end of the interview, because I was enjoying the family and feeling affectionate feelings toward them, it was natural for me to hug the members of the family. Just after I hugged the mother and went to the two sisters, I heard a little snickering by the two boys, aged eighteen and twelve. What crossed my mind was that these two boys were at a period where it might be awkward for them to engage in this kind of thing, even though I felt they wanted some kind of expression of affection from me. When I turned to the first of them, I commented that I had heard the snickering and that maybe this was a bit much for them, but I wanted them to know that I had these feelings. Then I gave them each an extra-warm handshake and a pat on the shoulder, trying to respect where they were at that point and at the same time to convey my message. What was interesting also was that the father was the last one I went to; I had the feeling that he was almost standing in line waiting and would be willing to hug but couldn't quite ask. When I made the overture to him, he came readily to be hugged. I know that men very often have had experiences in the past where it wasn't manly to have such feelings, and so I found myself telling the father that Bob Hope had spoken so many years ago about an individual who "had not been cuddled and so he curdled." This helped the father to put an acceptable face on this display of affection.

The observers watching the family yesterday could see life begin to be much more evident in these people. I am aware, right now, that when I think about my treatment sessions, I think of them as experiences in human contact which for me, without being in any sense mystical, create a feeling that I have had a journey and an adventure with other live beings. I hope that as a result of our journey, the people are feeling more alive, more lovable, more hopeful, more creative—and are seeing new ways to use themselves and to connect with each other. Often, I see people only one time. My hope is that every interview will result in a new window for each person to look through—with the result of feeling better about himself or herself and gaining the ability to do things more creatively with other members of his or her family. This is really what I mean by saying that I am dealing with a coping process rather than a problem-solving process.

I would like to return to my use of the communication stances as aids to developing changes in the coping process. I mentioned the four stances, which I expect to see in some combination, with all of the people who are experiencing problems in coping. Placating, blaming, being super-reasonable, and being irrelevant all appeared in yesterday's family. Incidentally, one of the things I have become increasingly conscious of is that the American dream about what a person should be really fits my category of the super-reasonable response. This response is: "For goodness sake, don't show any feeling!" This to me is sad, but it is also true.

At this point I will digress a moment and state that the stances are not rigid and unchangeable. Each of these ways of communicating can be renovated. If you are handling your responses by placating, one of the ravages going on within you is that you keep giving yourself messages that you don't count for very much. However, if you know how, you can renovate this ability to be tender, and bring it into your awareness, instead of just feeling an automatic given that you always have to please everyone.

Renovated blaming becomes your ability to stand up for yourself. Everyone needs to be able to do that, but you must do it realistically and consciously rather than automatically. Renovated super-reasonableness becomes the creative use of your intelligence. Using your intelligence is delightful; but if it is used only to protect yourself, it becomes rather boring and unfulfilling. Renovated irrelevancy becomes your ability to be spontaneous and to give yourself a new direction in awareness and in reality.

In any case, in dealing with a super-reasonable person like the father in yesterday's family, the therapist faces a most difficult problem. Super-reasonable people sit very still and upright; they move their faces very little, their voices are usually in a monotone, and they always talk very reasonably. You get this feeling of a kind of drying-up about the person; he or she is all locked in. As it happened, the father had been a Fundamentalist minister, and he had strong feelings about what was right and wrong. I noticed that he responded to all my overtures—the handshake, the questions, and the statements I made—in the same way. I felt that he listened, but I wasn't always sure he understood. I did find, and continue to find that people who organize their responses in this fashion use lots of words to say things. It is important for me to try to tune in wherever I can in a way that is going to touch the person. And so when someone is organized by using big words and being reasonable, it is natural for me to come in on that level.

Oftentimes therapists get bored by people who talk a lot. However, I need to have them talk enough so that I can understand what they are saying on the meta level. In the case of this man, he had told me about his repeated efforts to do what he wanted to do and how they continued to fail. Again, this was said in his dry, rather matter-of-fact voice. As I listened to him, I became aware that it sounded as though he had stopped trying. I asked him what had happened to his dreams. It sounded a little to me as if he had given up on his dreams. I began to see a light come into his eyes. The bottom half of his face didn't change particularly, but his eyes became a little wider and there was a little light in them. As I listened to his response, he said it was true; that he didn't have any more dreams. They were dead.

In my mind, I now pictured him in a sculpture—a lifeless inner body with an outer hard shell. I use these stances and ways of communicating, that I hear and see in my mind, as my guidelines to the kinds of interventions I make with people. If this is done in a trusting, understanding, hearing context, then new understandings emerge. By the end of yesterday's interview, the husband's whole face was beginning to respond, not just his eyes. I might say here—I think it is true of me and of others, too—that when I am listening to somebody, I am also looking at him or her and am aware of all his or her moving parts. I am aware of all the changes that may be going on. I am listening with my full self, with all of my senses.

There is another important element that I would like to mention. I call it the energy field. I think it is important because it goes along with touching. Around any well-integrated person there is a circular field that is about three feet in diameter. At the edge of this field, you can feel vibrations—at least I can! These vibrations are like unacknowledged territorial lines around the person. When a person is relatively well put-together, those lines feel like elastic. When you come up to them, first of all, you can physically feel them; you can feel that you are bumping against something. If it feels elastic, you know that you are there and that maybe you can reach over. I respect these lines. That's why I stay at arm's length. If I go closer to a person, I have already experimented as to whether or not his or her boundary will let me in. There seems to be a relation between the development of trust and the elasticity of this boundary.

When I am dealing with people who are very, very much out of contact with themselves, their energy field is only about two or three inches in diameter. I have to go a long way before I can feel any kind of vibration at all. It is a kind of deadness. I am virtually face to face with them before I get any kind of feeling of presence at all. When people have very violent insides, their field extends to about six feet—and I am very aware of that. We tend to overuse the word vibrations; but I know what that energy field feels like, and I am very respectful of that boundary. It is imaginary, but I can feel it in my body. When I'm around people in whom there is a lot of violence, I never go close until I can begin to feel the elasticity. I don't know if I am explaining this suitably, but it is a little like using your body to determine how far you can go. This is very relevant to the whole touching business because my touching doesn't take place unless I know that the other person's boundary is elastic.

Sight is also apart of this. The distance at which you can see someone—really see him—is probably nine or ten feet. At ten feet the outlines are there; the nuances are not. You can see fairly well at six feet; at about three feet you can see much better. I want to get to where I can be seen and heard as soon as I can. The process of going close is many times also the process of connecting—the slow way. You can't judge this by what you should do; you have to judge it by the way you feel. Some people who watched me work with a family and saw me touch said, "Aha! I see! All you have to do is touch." My answer was that touch has to be used just as carefully with people as with a hot stove. You are quite literally feeling your way. This is one of the reasons that, when I work with therapists and train them, I try to train their body awareness. For example, when people get into murderous rages, it helps me to be in a position of helping but yet not crowding. I don't think the touch connection works in that kind of situation. Perhaps some of you have noticed that when someone is in a rage and you touch him or her, you might get hit. The hit is not because the person wants to kill you (although he or she could) but because, at that time, the boundaries have been violated.

I wondered then about the other members of yesterday's family—and their dreams. For a few moments we talked about dreams that had not come to life. The wife's dream was of being able to have a life with her husband different from the one she had. She said she had started her marriage by always trying to please her husband. That had been what she was taught to do. She was now tired of it. I asked her if she would be willing to make a little picture with me. She agreed. I asked her to get down on her knees and to look up at her husband, whom I asked to stand on a stool. Then I asked the wife if what she was doing felt like anything she had ever felt before. She said that it did but she didn't want it to be like that anymore. Then I asked her husband how he felt up there, and he said he didn't like her being down there and he didn't like being on top. Then I asked them to fix it so they would both be comfortable. Of course, they ended up being eye-to-eye, both on the same level. It was following this that some expressions of hope began to appear on their faces.

What I want to emphasize here is that if I hear a person handling his or her responses in a super-reasonable fashion, I tune in at the level of the intellect but in such a way as to give the person an experience of really being heard and seen. If I shift to a person who, like yesterday's wife, is placating, I try to get in touch with what she hoped for herself and lead her to talk about some of her yearnings and loneliness. The wife did this, but it wouldn't have appeared unless I had asked.

With blamers, like the second oldest child, I have to get in touch with the longing to be connected. This was my approach yesterday when, rather than dealing with all the hate feelings, we focused instead on her own feelings about herself and her wish to be connected with her mother. What I found myself doing in each case was trying to help the person to stabilize. Sometimes I did this with a touch of my hand, or perhaps just by getting the person to be physically still for a moment in order to focus.

This is important to share with you because, as I sit with a family, my body tells me a great deal about where those people are and where their boundaries are. For example, the boundary is very, very close around a super-reasonable person. This is probably one of the reasons people say that the super-reasonable person is not "available." The boundary around an irrelevant person is all broken; you can't tell where it is. The boundary around a blamer is very far out and jagged. The placater is a very interesting person. His boundary is made out of liquid—out of whipped cream that is beginning to melt. It is there, but you can't tell much from it. Even though this is a somewhat picturesque way of talking about a person and his presence, it is something of which I am very aware, and I honor it. Perhaps a poetic way of putting it is this: What you are feeling at any point in time is how much of a person's life is willing to make itself known, with that fear, with that protectiveness. If you want to connect with that, you must be able to respect it.

My hands are my most valuable treatment asset. So are my body and my skin, in sensing what is going on; and my eyes in seeing; and the connections that all of these make. Hands are so important! This is one of the reasons I try to help people to educate their hands. Something else I do in affectional relationships with people is to help them to educate their bodies and also to be aware of space and boundaries. I am quite convinced that that's what this business of making connections really means. What I have just said helps me make a definition of intimacy. It is simply the freedom to respect the spaces between people—to go in when there is an invitation, and not to invade when there isn't one. That is real intimacy.

People often ask me, "How long is an interview?" It is as long as is necessary to make it possible to find and open a new window for people to look through. An interview can last anywhere from two to three hours. I am not doing office practice any more; when I was, I had three hours as my minimum time for an initial interview. I wanted people to leave the interview with something new that they could experiment with and live with. This means they go out of my office with a new awareness that they can use. It can be small or big, but that awareness carries with it some kind of hope—the hope that they can do something different about themselves, that life can be different for them in some way.

I timed the ensuing sessions to occur whenever another step was readying itself. This pattern is not rigid. My thought is that every interview has a life of its own. Nothing says that I am going to be around tomorrow to see you again or that you are going to be around. I work toward a new possibility and we have a closing on something as the family and I leave each other. That does not mean that all the work is finished. It never means that, because we can go on growing forever. But it does mean, that at the end of the interview, we have something new that can be useful.

For example, with the family I saw yesterday, the ending for me was my telling them that I enjoyed being with them and being a part of their life for two hours; and that I would have really liked to have been able to continue to be a part, but my life needs didn't make that possible. If by chance we were to meet again, I would like it very much. The idea is that an interview has a life of its own and the next interview will have still another life. Because if you are really growing, each interview will have still another life. Because if you are really growing, each interview is totally different. People are in different places and the therapist is in a different place. At any rate, that is how I like to look at it.

The promise I make to people is that I will tell them everything I can and show them everything I can. I cannot promise that I will tell all that is in me because I do not know that. I can tell you only what I know is there. Many of you who are reading may hear things that I never intended, but that may be there anyway. My hope for you is that maybe you have found some new windows. Just as I did with the family yesterday, I have tried here to open some doors for you. I hope it will be useful.

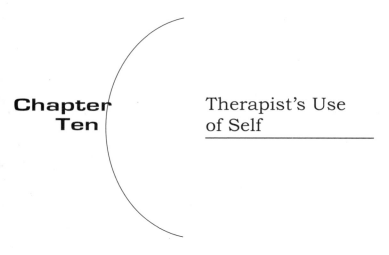

Chapter Ten

Therapist's Use of Self

Introduction by Carl Sayles

In this article Virginia Satir challenges therapist's to work experientially with families, modeling the relationship between the therapist, family, and the process. She brilliantly points out the various places where the process can be deepened by observing, not only what is taking place with the client family, but also being aware of the process going on inside the therapist. She notes the significance of the therapist's own body posture, tone, energy level, and positioning in comparison to the family.

A therapist working in process with an individual, couple or family, needs to develop a deepening sense of his or her own awareness of communication patterns. Without this deepening awareness a therapist can block the therapeutic process, possibly stopping it without knowing or understanding how or why it happened. The effect of this lack of awareness can be a cutting off of the very process that has taken time and energy to nurture and develop. To keep the process moving, the awareness of the therapist needs to remain sharp and ever present to changes in the therapeutic dynamic while honoring each person and their process.

In this work, a therapist is not only unraveling an old process and way of being, but is also helping to build a new one that is stronger and healthier. A therapist who is aware of her or his own external and internal processes can better understand and reflect on where each person might be in their process, thereby enhancing the experience for each person in the family system, whether *the family is present or not. The effect of this enhancement is that individuals begin to take more personal responsibility for themselves. Overall, people begin to feel better about being a part of the larger extended system because they feel like they matter.*

Considering that much of what Satir unfolds in this article is what is being taught today, it is an excellent exploration into some of the "how-to" of using self reflectively and not getting caught in the trap of moving too far or too fast into the client's world. Whether working with individuals, couples or families, the use of self as a reflective tool is the same. The ultimate goal is to help therapists, new and seasoned, explore how they might use their own experience of the therapeutic interaction taking place to bring about a deeper level of meaning and potential change for the person in process.

■ ■ ■

The most difficult aspect of family therapy is that the therapist is operating on many different levels simultaneously. This principle of simultaneity may seem overwhelming as we discuss it here. However, we would like to say to beginning family therapists that the ability to operate on all of these levels at the same time does develop with time and experience. The problem is that the beginning therapist must be prepared to lose families without being harsh with himself. He may be operating very well on one or more levels, but miss another important one, which will lose him the family in treatment. It is simply impossible to become proficient enough on all of these levels all at once. Therefore, the beginning family therapist does not have the means to flow freely with the family's energy and process. At this point, we would like to enumerate the major simultaneous levels of operation.

The therapist must be in and out of the family system at the same time. The therapist operates best by taking enough physical distance from the family so that he can see the entire family within his area of vision. He watches the family's interaction and communication patterns. In addition, he tunes into his own experience of sitting in with the family system. For example, a therapist is interviewing a family with both parents and five children. He is sitting between the two parents. The interaction of the family members seems to be moving fairly freely verbally, but they are getting nowhere. The therapist looks at their patterns and considers the possibility that they may be masking the real problem by trying to cover too much ground. So, he asks them to take a specific incident that occurred recently and go into it in detail in terms of what each person's picture was, what each said and felt. They begin to do this and all seem to be involved but, again, the feeling tone of the session has the quality of spinning wheels or bogging down. The therapist then momentarily checks out of the system and into his insides. He picks up a heavy feeling, a chaotic feeling, and he is also aware that he feels more and more constricted as he sits between the two parents. He offers all of this information to the family; thus intervening back into the system in an attempt to shake it up because all the data indicates that the family is not dealing with the real issues. The family responds to the therapist's observations with confusion on the part of the parents, and nods of understanding from the children.

The therapist then asks each child in turn to change places with him, sit between the parents, and communicate his feelings about this experience. Each child communicates either by his words or his physical behavior that this is an uncomfortable place to be. The therapist then offers to the parents that six people, including himself, are picking up something that is transpiring between them. He then asks what each of them is experiencing. He checks in with his own insides and realizes he is much relieved and the heaviness has vanished. This data is validated by the system as the physical behavior and energy level in the family is much less constricted. Therefore, he knows he is in pay dirt. He then asks the parents to face each other and begin to explore what might be going on between them.

As the parents take physical positions facing each other and looking at each other directly, the tension again builds. The therapist is aware of his hands perspiring; he checks out the other family members and they are fidgeting, withdrawing or interrupting in some way. He uses this data to again move back into the system to keep it open. He offers his observation, and wonders if they are frightened or worried. Two of the children say that they are but are unable to clarify the reasons for their feelings. Both parents confirm that they are very tense. The therapist asks them to describe their tension to each other. As you can see, the therapist is constantly moving into the system with interventions designed to break all the rules and trigger crises in the system, in order to develop movement. At the same time, he keeps checking back into his own internal system for data about the family, since they are so well defended and therefore unrevealing in their external image. When he gets data from his internal processes that is incongruent or discrepant with the family's image, he looks for behavior or communication patterns that would support or deny his internal data. When he gets supportive behavior, he puts pressure on the family to further explore along whatever pathway produces that anxiety.

In this particular family, it came out over time that everyone in the family was operating as though he or she had many secrets from the others. The parents were involved in husband-and-wife-swapping encounters, which they thought the children didn't know about. The husband and wife each had had brief periodic affairs that each thought were unknown to the other. The children often lied to their parents and thought they were getting away with it. What emerged as these things came out was that all of these things were known by all family members, but never discussed, as though they were all in a conspiracy of pretense. The result was a buildup of tremendous rage and frustration, which was producing a fear and distance in the family.

In another instance, the therapist who is working with a judgmental family will suddenly find himself in an argument with the father in the family about who is right. If the part of himself that is outside the system is operating, he will become aware that he has been caught by the system and can offer this to the family. "Look, here I am doing the same thing you do to each other; I'm arguing about who is right or wrong, instead of sharing my feelings and dealing with yours. That's a statement to me about how strong your system is and how difficult it must be for each of you to break out of that framework, even though it isn't working for you any longer."

The therapist must also be aware of his own body posture, his tone, and his energy level in comparison with the family. It is important that he be discrepant with the system. Otherwise, if he is the same as the system, he will support and reinforce its negative processes. For example, the family appears very depressed and heavy. The therapist finds himself working hard to put energy into the system and he feels increasingly heavy and depressed. If he allows this to continue, he will become angry and withdraw or attack the family, or he will feel guilty because nothing is happening, and work even harder.If, on the other hand, he is able to step out of the system, e can observe what is happening to him as a message about the system. Then he can say to the family: "As I work with you, I find my voice getting lower and lower, my posture sinking, and my gut feeling depressed as though it is my fault you aren't producing or moving or getting what you want. I wonder if that is the message you perceive from one another?" He then throws his data back into the system, which is a clear message that he can maintain his boundaries and therefore can help them in a way that leaves him intact, and them responsible for their own choices. That is something they are not able to do with each other. So, he is operating in opposition to the negative processes in the family system, and at the same time is modeling a positive process for opening and exploring, because he is using himself to observe and comment without criticizing or depreciating any of them.

The therapist is constantly checking back and forth between his own inferences, in terms of assessment and treatment direction, with the salient processes emerging in the family's interactional flow. For example, as he is interviewing a family in a first session, he observes that the interaction is limited. Family members do not touch each other or look at each other when they talk. Their body postures are stiff and rigid; the dress of all the family members is noticeably discrepant from the one member whom all others identify as the patient or the disturbed one in the family. Verbally, the focus is on this member—the son, for example, and his use of drugs. The underlying message is that the family would be fine if he were not around and he would be fine if he had never known about drugs. The father lectures as though he were on a soapbox when he talks, usually looking at the ceiling or out at some unknown audience. The mother is passive in her behavior, does not speak unless drawn out and then responds in a tiny, little girl voice. The daughter lectures like the father, appears more the wife in the family than the mother does. The family sits in such a way that the son seems to be outside the system.

The therapist notes all these factors and begins to make inferences in his head about possible meanings and direction that may go something like this: There seems to be a role dysfunction between mother and daughter in that daughter appears more the adult. That, coupled with the mother's passive behavior and her little girl voice, suggests that the mother doesn't have much to give as an adult woman; and the family, including the husband, is not getting any nurturing from her even though she may perform as a very capable homemaker. That suggests a serious breakdown between the parents in terms of giving and receiving, which seems validated by the husband's stiffness, deadness and the total feeling of asexuality that the family projects.

The therapist further infers that this has been a long standing problem in view of the rigidity of the roles and the family's defense system, so he cannot push the marital relationship prematurely. Therefore, perhaps the best direction to go is to open up the communication between father and son. The son is the one most discrepant with the system and therefore perhaps most available to change, and the father is so desperate about loss of control over his son that he might be amenable to some change. The therapist decides he must move slowly because the family is obviously very frightened and could panic and become overwhelmed easily. He is about to proceed in this direction when suddenly the wife lashes out at her husband, "I'm sick of your preaching and your judgments about how everyone should be! I don't blame Jimmy for getting out! If it weren't for the children I would kill myself."

At this point, the evolving process is making it clear that the therapist has to shift both in his inference process and his treatment direction. That doesn't mean that his previous inferences were incorrect, necessarily. It does mean that the mother is in crisis, that crisis is the most salient factor in the family's current energy flow and, therefore, it has to be dealt with immediately. If the therapist does not deal with this crisis, but proceeds with his previous inferences, the family will assume he is not able to handle them and will not trust him. In order to build trust, the therapist always has to go where the energy—the aliveness, the feeling—in the system is. Again that is discrepant with the dysfunctional system, which is dysfunctional because family members are afraid of their aliveness (intensity) and do not know how to handle it without hurting themselves or others. It is the therapist's job to teach them how to handle their energy in ways that promote growth and do not result in internal loss or damage.

The therapist's inference level shifts, the mother feels pushed beyond her support system; she is potentially suicidal. The message in her words, behavior, tone, and body position, is congruent: panic and desperation. The therapist acknowledges that she is obviously in terrible pain, and asks that she share more of this pain with the family. He asks family members to listen without feeling as though they are responsible, but just hear and stay in touch with their own feelings so that they can share them.

As the mother opens up more, the therapist may move in either of two directions, depending on where the energy is. If it appears that the wife is wanting support and release of feelings with her family, he will move in an interactional direction; helping her to come out with her feelings in a way that doesn't blame, dump or depreciate others, and enabling others in the family to learn how to hear and respond with their own feelings. If, on the other hand, her panic and rage seem to be out of control, he infers that it is vital to give her some release or she may suffer a serious depression or make a suicide attempt. Therefore, he moves in the direction of a physical release through Gestalt techniques like beating a chair and screaming. This would be supported with much explanation, encouragement, and understanding offered to her and the rest of the family so that they can tolerate and allow this shift.

When she is relieved, the therapist would then integrate this change into the system by getting everyone else's reaction—both to her and within themselves—and then teaching them to look at this explosion in a growth framework, while at the same time supporting how frightened all of them must be. He would explain that, even though they are fearful of change, they are faced with the reality that their old ways of operating are killing them, as evidenced by the son's symptom and the mother's feelings expressed in the session. Therefore, in order to live and grow, they have to change. Thus it is clear to them what their choices are - and that there are choices. The family is still in charge of what it does. The therapist does not take over. He then explains that he will assist the family in learning new ways of operating that fit them better and are not destructive, but it will take time. He may discuss with the family members what safety valves they will need in the meantime to give them temporary relief while they are learning new ways. His inference level tells him that the family members are very childlike, need a lot of support and structuring about what has happened to prevent a crisis during the week. There may be one anyway, no matter how much support they get, so the therapist is preparing for that by opening up and stating that this can happen and it isn't terrible. It just means that families have different learning patterns, and so it is important to explore how we can handle a crisis if it does occur, with minimal upset to the system.

The important point is that the therapist does make inferences continually, as a way of cataloguing and assimilating all the data constantly in front of him. But he must also be prepared to shift instantly if the flow of energy in the family system moves to a new or different level.

The therapist must be aware of communication patterns among the family members, between himself and the family as a whole, and between himself and each family member. He may observe that, although family members say father is the boss in the family, mother seems to be the spokesman. Mother and father often don't speak to each other directly; they speak through the oldest son, who translates to each what the other one means. This is discrepant with the family members' insistence that they all communicate easily with each other, except for the daughter whom they see as the family "problem." All family members, except for the daughter, communicate with the therapist with a deferent manner, as though he is a judge or some superior being. Yet, they do not accept any feedback that he offers them. They are quick to defend, explain or give reasons why what he offers isn't so, and they don't allow themselves any room to assimilate and consider what he says. It is as though they are so couched for defense that they don't even hear him. No one is open to any feedback that suggests change, because they see feedback as criticism and attack. The father in the family is wary even of supportive, empathetic comments from the therapist. The mother is more amenable to warmth from the therapist, but the children quickly interfere if it looks as though the therapist and the mother may be developing a positive connection.

In this instance, the communication patterns on all these levels seem to give a congruent message: The family members are all feeling emotionally hungry and depleted. Everyone wants, but no one feels he is getting anything. People in the family do not listen, cannot accept feedback and are not yet ready for a therapy contract. Their beginning sessions would be geared toward a slow, supportive explanation of what is involved in therapy and what their alternatives are separate from therapy, so that they can make a decision about what they want. The therapist would handle this preparation phase with recognition of their immediate sense of helplessness and emotional drain. The family may or may not be at a point where they can actually move into therapy. But it will be a therapeutic experience for them to be clearly confronted, in a nonjudgmental way, with the real issues they are facing and their possible choices about these issues. That process alone is discrepant with their own way of dealing with each other, which is critical and demanding.

In another family, there might be considerable discrepancy among the communication patterns, which would require a very different way of handling the family system. When these family members talk to each other, their words may express denial of their feeling, but when they talk to the therapist, the feelings may begin to emerge. The therapist could then use that phenomenon to explore with family members what they experience with him that they would like to have with each other, so that they could share and communicate.

In still another situation, there may be coalitions. Father can communicate with daughter and mother, but not with son. If he can also communicate with a male therapist, then the therapist might assume there is a learning gap in his experience in the area due to an absent or unknown father, and explore that possibility with him. If he cannot communicate with the therapist, but is withholding and distant, the therapist might assume that there are some feelings of hurt and rage connected with his father, which are in the way. He can then explore his boyhood relation-ship with his dad in terms of what he got that he didn't want or what he wanted that he didn't get.

We think that the most important area of observation for the therapist has to do with body and behavioral clues. There are numerous simultaneous levels of observation around this data. We think the most important are:

1. The congruency of the body messages of each member of the family with his words, tone, and quality of expression. The father's whole organism may express a congruent message of rigidity and containment. Or, his body message may express rigidity but be discrepant with his voice and facial expression, which indicate that he is close to tears. The therapist notes the father's congruency or discrepancy of expression and also observes the reaction of each of the other family members to this expression from father.

2. The therapist's own body posture is important as a way of assessing the family system. The therapist may be slumping in an increasingly depressed position as he works with the family. He may be sitting with arms and legs crossed—a possible statement that either he or the family, or both, are trying to

go in two directions at once. The point is, it is helpful if the therapist can be aware of his own body posture, both on the level of what it may express about the family with whom he is working as well as the level of what it means in relation to his own personal circumstances at the moment.

3. The therapist must be aware of the discrepancy of body movement to the family system. For example, a family may be discussing its situation very reasonably, but there are constant body movements that seem to just ripple through the system from one family member to another.

4. Body movements may occur in patterns. For example, each time the communication gets to a feeling level between the parents, the youngest son starts kicking the table. Or, every time father starts to become angry, the children begin stretching and yawning. The therapist then codes these patterns for intervention at an appropriate point.

The most important tools the therapist has are his own internal manifestations, as they relate to all these other levels we've been describing. If his internal experience of the interview is different from all the other data he is observing, and he is fairly sure his reaction is not related to something going on in his own life, then the most effective way to proceed is on the basis of that internal data. The beginning therapist will usually not do this because he doesn't feel he has educated himself enough to his internal manifestations to be sure of them. So, he will try all other directions first, but will usually end up back with his internal experience. This is all right because it takes time and experience for the therapist to test out his resources in this respect until he feels they are finely tuned and balanced. However, once he is more sure of himself in this area, he will save himself and the family considerable treatment time.

The therapist may learn via checking out his internal manifestations with the family that, when he feels tension in his stomach, he is picking up fear. When he feels a pain through his neck and shoulders, he is perceiving anger. When he becomes sleepy, even though he has had sufficient sleep, he is experiencing rage. Everyone is different in terms of how his body reacts to subliminal feeling messages, and each person must learn to read his own clues. However, if the therapist takes the trouble to learn about himself in this way, he will never be at a loss for an alternative way to proceed in a therapy session. When all else fails, this mechanism is always reliable.

In addition to all of the above, the therapist also operates as an observer, a camera, a sex and communication model—and he determines the degree of intimacy to which the family will go with one another and with him. As an observer, it is important for the therapist to learn how to look and see without interpretation, just for registration, and to teach the family to do the same. Many of us have not learned just how to simply observe. For example, a therapist may ask a couple to sit facing each other, look at each other and say what they see. The wife looks at the husband and instead of saying, "His eyes are blue, his skin is tan and smooth," she will say, "He looks angry at me." That is an interpretation, not an observation.

Many times in the process of training family therapists at the institute, we will ask a therapist just to observe a family and tell us what he sees. We often get comments like, "They are frightened of each other and the therapy situation," when the observable data is, "The family members do not look at each other or the therapist, they look down at the floor. The body postures of family members appear tight and closed with legs crossed, arms folded and shoulders hunched." Frequently, we will turn off the sound in a video tape of a family and teach people to just comment on what they observe happening without interpretation or judgment. Learning how to observe is a basic step in becoming a family therapist and a basic step in developing intimacy in a family. The therapist operates as a camera in that he captures data from communication patterns, interactional processes and other observable phenomena for development into his internal picture of how the family operates. What are the negative processes they use for relating? How do these processes occur, and what results do they produce that are destructive to the family. He uses his eyes and ears to perceive what happens when family members try to reach each other, and what breaks down in their attempts to make contact. He mirrors their behavior as though he were actually taking a picture of it. He may express this by imitating the family communication patterns, by getting involved in the system and commenting on what that is like for him, or by sharing his picture of how he, as an outsider, sees the family operating.

The therapist is a model of sexuality in terms of the way he communicates himself to the family and the way in which he responds to the family. If a male/female co-therapy team is operating, then this factor becomes even more important, because the therapy itself depends on their ability to communicate clearly and constructively with each other. Family members get confronted with all their mythology about male and female roles. They learn that feelings are not male or female, they are just feelings. Men and women both can be tender, powerful, sensitive, petty, warm, considerate or overbearing; there are no feelings peculiar to one sex and not the other. In addition, they learn that ways of expressing feelings are not distinctly male or female. Men and women both can cry, rage, get hysterical, have temper tantrums, express helplessness or power, and it has nothing to do with whether they are male or female, strong or weak. Having feelings and learning how to express them in ways appropriate to one's own unique nature is just part of being human.

If the female therapist sees the husband's expression of anger at her (the therapist) as a desire to make contact, or his ability to express tears as a strength, she models for the wife a new way of perceiving as well as a different way of responding to her husband. If the male therapist hears the wife's criticism of him without having to defend himself or convince her otherwise—but can respond to her nonverbal behavior which is expressing pain—he models that for the husband. He shows him how to be in charge of himself and not use his wife as judge, as well as how to respond to more than one level of communication.

The degree of intimacy that a family will pursue in its growth in therapy is determined by the degree of intimacy with which the therapist is comfortable. The family tests this out in terms of their relationship with him (the therapist), and their relationships with each other. In the beginning phases of treatment, family members will test out whether the therapist is in charge of himself. Can he do with them what he is asking them to do with each other: to be honest and open about his feelings in ways that are not judgmental or deprecating? Sometimes a family will produce an uproar situation, and it is important that the therapist be able to take charge of himself and the situation by setting his own boundaries in terms of the conditions he requires for working. He must do this in a way that leaves the family in charge of themselves, so that they do not feel as though the therapist is treating them like infants.

Sometimes families feel very grateful to a therapist and want to love him by asking personal questions, expressing thanks and appreciation, or touching him. It the therapist has difficulty receiving affection from people, he may block such expression with interpretations that the family is being seductive with him to avoid something in their process, or with curt responses, or by simply not acknowledging what the family is doing and shifting to their interaction. What the therapist needs to understand is that he is not just tearing down old processes that are destructive to the family; he is also helping them build new ones that will enhance their experience with each other. Allowing them to give to him is a way of teaching them how to do this with each other. In some families parents can give to their children, but they do not know how to allow the children to give to them. Many people have difficulty receiving, and the therapist can be an important model in this respect by learning how to genuinely enjoy a family's ability to give to him.

In our teaching of therapists, we have become aware that many people have difficulty when working with couples who have gone beyond their problem areas and are moving into deepening their intimacy with each other. It is not infrequent that a couple will be in a beautiful flow of interaction and the therapist will interrupt with an interpretation, completely oblivious that he has just cut off the very process he has spent months trying to develop with this couple. When we brought this to the therapist's attention and explored with him what might be going on, we found that the couple's deepening intimacy has triggered feelings of loneliness or dissatisfaction on the part of the therapist, or that the couple is going into a depth the therapist has not experienced and does not know how to handle. Our experience has been that therapists who are skilled in techniques and processes can help people develop and express all kinds of feelings that the therapist himself may not be in touch with within himself. However, when it comes to building a relationship, we find that the therapist cannot take people where he has not been. This doesn't mean that he should stop working in these areas; it simply means that he must be aware of his current stage of growth and thus aware when the family he is working with has gone beyond him. This is not in any way a criticism of the therapist. We are all in varying stages of growth all the time and usually the kind of clients with whom we work best will change as we develop. We will find ourselves working with different types of problems and relationships at different stages of our own growth.

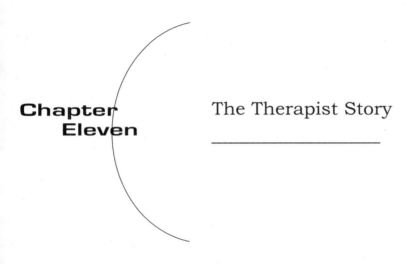

Chapter Eleven

The Therapist Story

Introduction by Moira Haagen

Imagine for a moment.... You are a beautiful Stradivarius violin, finely tuned and well cared for. The instant your strings are touched, beautiful music pours forth. It builds and swells to a crescendo, touching and inspiring all those around you. They are filled with joy and hope, and their life force wants to dance along. How encouraging and empowering that might be!

In The Therapist Story, which Virginia Satir published in 1987, a year before her death, she presents those of us who are therapists with an opportunity to experience such fulfillment by exploring how we can impact the therapeutic process and outcomes for our clients through our own use of self—the main tool for facilitating change. She beautifully illustrates this through her metaphorical description of the musical instrument for a therapist's use of self. Our clients present the music, and how well we understand and hear that music depends on how well we care for ourselves, how well we are tuned into ourselves, and how competent we are at our work.

Amidst the growing research and attention given to the nature of the human being in medicine, science and technology, Satir expresses awareness of a new consciousness that places a high value on being human. She highlights how our understanding of human behavior has evolved and how the nature of the therapeutic relationship has been redefined, placing these changes in the history of Freud's psychoanalysis through to holistic and existential approaches. Satir's work constantly both insists upon and exemplifies the centrality of the therapist-client relationship—of a self interacting with a self, and the inevitable and mutual impact the therapist and client have on each other as human beings. It parallels closely what Martin Buber described as the "I-Thou" relationship.

In this climate of change, she invites us to focus our attention on the ways in which the therapist's use of self can be of positive value in treatment. Central to this invitation is Satir's rich discussion of a therapist's use of power, how that power is a function of the self of the therapist, and how therapists have the choice to use that power to influence therapeutic results positively or negatively. She reminds us of our vulnerability as human beings, that making contact with our clients is so much more than the theories or techniques alone, that each client is not just "a trophy on the therapist's success ladder."

In The Therapist Story, we can experience a fresh and encouraging opportunity to look at how well we hear and understand the music our clients present. As therapists in our process of becoming, we need to take care of ourselves as if we were hand-crafted violins, keeping ourselves well-tuned and ready to play on the stage of life.

■ ■ ■

Freud's contributions have radically altered our thinking about psychotherapy and human behavior. Although this has resulted in the development of many theories and techniques of therapy, the basic ingredient remains the relationship between the therapist and the patient. Since the latter comes to the former in a state of need, the therapist holds enormous power, which can be used negatively for exploitation and manipulation, or positively for healing and growth. The potential for the abuse of such power makes the value system and beliefs of the therapist vitally important. By being congruent, the therapist can create a context of trust and caring, which enables the patient to dispel his or her fears and begin to explore new growth patterns. Therapy is a deeply intimate and vulnerable experience, requiring sensitivity to one's own state of being as well as to that of the other. It is the meeting of the deepest self of the therapist with the deepest self of the patient or client.

One hundred years ago, as today, we were nearing a new century. Then as now, people strongly felt that they lived in a period of great change. America was moving from a predominantly rural, agricultural way of life to an urban, industrial culture. The battle for human rights was emerging. Unions were forming to protect the rights of workers. Concerned citizens were lobbying for protection of children through child labor laws. Social reformers were mounting campaigns for women's suffrage. In the sciences, foundations were being laid for today's nuclear weaponry, space travel and electronic communications. In that same period a new psychology was being formulated that would change the way we think about ourselves. I would like to think that the advent of another new century will bring with it another change of consciousness about ourselves that places a high value on humanness. The therapist who makes self an essential factor in the therapeutic process is a herald of that new consciousness.

Sigmund Freud opened his practice one hundred years ago in Vienna. In 1921, he visited the United States, bringing with him the new form of psychotherapy which he called psychoanalysis. His main thesis was that human beings carry the seeds of their construction, as well as their destruction, within them. This was a radical idea that eventually initiated a revolutionary breakthrough in mental health practice. Up to that time, the prevailing reasons for deviant and other unacceptable forms of behavior were thought to be bad environment, personal unworthiness, and "genetic taint." The cure was usually isolation, punishment, abandonment, or death.

Freud's views also offered a new way of understanding human behavior. By 1940, psychoanalytic concepts underlaid almost all psychological thinking and treatment; and it continued that way until the appearance of existential and holistic thinking in the 60s. In some ways, I compare the impact of Freudian concepts with the work of Jellinek (1960), who advanced the idea that alcoholism was a disease and not the result of perversity or weakness. That, too, changed society's way of thinking and eventually led to new methods of treatment that offered hope to those who previously had no hope.

Originally, psychoanalytic treatment was administered by a trained psychotherapist (usually a physician) who, by "analyzing" the emotional experience and process of the patient, hoped to clear the way for the growth of health within the troubled individual. The early treatment model was that of the traditional doctor-patient relationship. The aim of treatment then, as it is today, was the eradication of symptoms, although the nature and meaning of symptoms have been greatly expanded over the years. The basic elements of psychotherapy remain the same, namely a therapist, a patient, a context, the interaction between the therapist and patient, and a model for approaching treatment. However, the definitions of these elements have also expanded and changed through additions and deletions over time. For example, the "patient" now is sometimes known as the "client," and may represent an individual, a group or a family (Rogers, 1951). The therapist may also be called a counselor, and can include one, two, or even more persons. The therapist may be drawn from a variety of disciplines in addition to medicine and psychiatry, such as psychology, social work, education or theology. The context now includes the office, the home, the hospital and the school.

The therapeutic interaction is also seen as a relationship between therapist and patient and may be characterized by a variety of treatment approaches, such as psychoanalysis, psychodrama, Gestalt therapy, transactional analysis, the various body therapies, family therapy and a host of others. The model of therapy has been expanded from the traditional, authoritarian doctor-patient relationship to include the patient as a partner (Hollender & Szasz, 1956).

We have all observed that two people using the same approach have come out with quite different results. We have also seen that two other people using quite different approaches can come out with similarly successful results. Yet very few training programs really deal with the person of the therapist. Those that do are usually in Psychoanalytic and Jungian Institutes where a training psychoanalysis is required, or in some family training programs.

The Role of Self in Therapy

Common sense dictates that the therapist and the patient must inevitably impact on one another as human beings. This involvement of the therapist's "self," or "personhood" occurs regardless of, and in addition to, the treatment philosophy or the approach. Techniques and approaches are tools. They come out differently in different hands. Because the nature of the relationship between therapist and patient makes the latter extremely vulnerable, it is incumbent upon the therapist to keep that relationship from being an exercise in the negative use of power or of developing dependency—both of which ultimately defeat therapeutic ends.

Freud recognized the power of the therapist. He maintained that the successful therapist had to handle his personal life in such a way as not to become entangled in the personal life of the patient. This led to the neutral, nonpersonal format of the psychoanalytic couch, with the therapist out of sight and relatively non-active; this despite the fact that Freud is reported to have given massage at times to his patients and to have become actively involved in their lives. Needleman (1985) claims that the secret of Freud's great success and creativity was due to the great force of his personal attention to his patients, which enabled him to project a quality of compassion and insight that radiated a healing influence.

Perhaps doubting his own capacity and that of others not to negatively influence patients, Freud developed the idea of mandatory training analysis for all psychotherapists, during which the trainees were supposed to understand and master their own conflicts and neuroses. This requirement was aimed at protecting the patient and creating the optimum conditions for change.

These ideas clearly stood on two basic principles: Therapists have the power to damage patients, and they are there to serve patients, not the other way around. Most therapists today would agree that they would not consciously want to harm their patients. On the contrary, they would claim that they try to create treatment contexts that are beneficial to their patients. Most therapists would also say that they are there to serve their patients. However, the words "harm" and "serve" are open to many interpretations.

Furthermore there was, and is, the idea that unconsciously, without malice or intent, therapists can harm patients through their own unresolved problems (Langs, 1985). One manifestation of this concept is reflected in what Freud called countertransference. Briefly, this means that therapists mistakenly and unconsciously see patients as sons, daughters, mothers or fathers, thereby projecting onto their patients something that does not belong—a real case of mistaken identity. This is a trap, well recognized by many therapists. However, unless therapists are very clear and aware, they may be caught in the trap without knowing it. Unless one knows what is going on, it is tempting to blame the patient for a feeling of being stuck as a therapist. Further manifestations of this phenomenon are rescuing or protecting, taking sides, or rejecting a patient, and, again, putting the responsibility on the patient.

When the prevailing model of therapeutic transaction, which is the authoritarian doctor-patient relationship, is experienced as one of dominance and submission, the patient and therapist can easily move into a power play that tends to reinforce childhood learning experiences. Throughout the therapeutic experience, the therapist may unwittingly replicate the negative learning experience of the patient's childhood and call it treatment. For instance when a therapist maintains that she knows when she doesn't know, she is modeling behavior similar to that of the patient's parent. The dominance and submission model increases chances for the therapist to live out her own ego needs for control. Manifestations of this control can appear to be benevolent, as in, "I am the one who helps you; therefore, you should be grateful," or malevolent, as in "You'd better do what I tell you, or I won't treat you." These, of course, are shades of childhood past. When they are present in therapy, treatment aims will be defeated.

Power and Therapy

The above are all disguised power issues. But, power has two faces: one is about controlling the other; the second is about empowering the other. The use of power is a function of the self of the therapist. It is related to the therapist's self-worth, which governs the way in which the therapist handles her ego needs.

Use of power is quite independent of any therapeutic technique or approach, although there are some therapeutic approaches that actually are based on the therapist maintaining a superior position (Dreikurs, 1960). There also are cases where there is outright and conscious exploitation by the therapist and some even justify their aggressive, sexual, or other unprofessional behavior on the grounds that it is beneficial to the patient (Langs, 1985). Once, a man came to my office with a bullwhip in his hand and asked me to beat him with it so he could become sexually potent. While I believed that it was possible that this method would work for him, I rejected it on the basis that it did not fit my values. I offered to help him in other ways and he accepted.

Using patients for one's own ego needs or getting them mixed up with one's own life is ethically unsound. However, the therapist can be in the same position as the patient—denying, distorting or projecting needs. It is possible for a patient or a client to activate something within the therapist of which the latter is unaware. It is easy to respond to a patient as though he or she is someone else in one's past or present, and if one is not aware that this is going on, it will needlessly complicate the situation. If one is a family therapist, it is likely that somewhere, at least once, one will see a family that duplicates some aspects of one's own family. When this happens and the therapist has not yet worked out the difficulties with his or her own family, the client may be stranded or misled because the therapist is also lost. Therapists should recognize that they are just as vulnerable as patients.

While therapists facilitate and enhance patients' ability and need to grow, they should at the same time be aware that they also have the ability and need. One way to avoid burn-out is to keep growing and learning. A great part of our behavior is learned from modeling, and therapists can model ways of learning and growing. It is also important to model *congruence*. An oversimplified definition of congruence is that one looks like one feels, says what one feels, and means and acts in accordance with what one says. Such congruence develops trust. This is the basis for the emotional honesty between therapist and patient, which is the key to healing. When a therapist says one thing and feels another, or demonstrates something that she denies, she is creating an atmosphere of emotional dishonesty that makes it an unsafe environment for the patient. I find that there is a level of communication beyond words and feelings, in which life communicates with life and understands incongruence. Young children show this awareness more easily. In adults, this level of communication usually presents itself in hunches or in vague feelings of uneasiness, or sensing. If I, as a therapist, am denying, distorting, projecting or engaging in any other form of masking, and am unaware of my own inner stirrings, I am communicating these to those around me no matter how well I think I am disguising them.

If patients feel that they are at risk because they feel "one down" in relation to the therapist, they will not report their distressed feelings and will develop defenses against the therapist. The therapist in turn, not knowing about this, can easily misunderstand the patient's response as resistance, instead of legitimate self-protection against the therapist's incongruence. Therapy is an intimate experience. For people to grow and change they need to be able to allow themselves to become open, which makes them vulnerable. When they are vulnerable, they need protection. It is the therapist's responsibility to create a context in which people feel and are safe, and this requires sensitivity to one's own state. For example, it is quite possible for a therapist who is focusing on a technique or a theoretical construct to be unaware that her own facial features and voice tone are conveying the messages to which the patient is responding.

The presence of resistance is a manifestation of fear, and calls for the utmost in honesty, congruence and trust on the part of the therapist. The only times that I have experienced difficulty with people are when I was incongruent. I either tried to be something I wasn't, or to withhold something I knew, or to say something I did not mean. I have great respect for that deep level of communication where one really knows when and whom one can trust. I think it comes close to what Martin Buber called the "I - Thou" relationship (Buber, 1970).

Very little change goes on without the patient and therapist becoming vulnerable. Therapists know that they have to go beyond patient defenses so that they can help them to become more open and vulnerable. Defenses are ways patients try to protect themselves when they feel unsafe. When the therapist acts to break down defenses, the therapeutic interaction becomes an experience that is characterized by, "who has the right to tell whom what to do, or who wins." In this struggle, the therapist, like the parent, has to win—and the patient loses.

When the patient is somehow thought of as a trophy on the therapist's success ladder, it is another repetition of the way in which many children experience their parents, where the children were expected to be a showcase for family values. Sometimes the therapist puts the patient in a position of being a pawn between two opposing authorities, as when a therapist puts a child between the parents, or between the parents and an institutional staff.

When the therapist sets out to help someone and leaves no doubt that she knows what is best for the patient, she is subjecting the patient to repetition of another childhood experience. There are those therapists who feel challenged to make something of the patient, "even if it kills you." These are often therapists who want to give messages of validation, although the outcomes are often very different.

The Positive Use of the Self

If the therapist can influence therapeutic results negatively through their use of the self, then it must be possible to use the self for positive results. The therapist has that power by virtue of her role and status and person. We know that this power can be misused and misdirected. However, the therapist also has the choice to use her power for empowering. Because the patient is vulnerable, the therapist also has the choice to use her power to empower patients towards their own growth.

In the new model of treatment that emerged in the 1950s and 1960s, the therapist began to form a partnership with the patient. Patient and therapist could work together utilizing their respective actions, reactions and interactions. The therapist was encouraged to model congruent behavior, and the focus of the therapeutic partnership was on developing health through working with the whole person. Eradication of the symptom was achieved by the development of a healthy state, which no longer required the symptom. (In the traditional, authoritarian, doctor-patient model, the emphasis was first on eradicating the symptom, with the hope that health would follow.)

When the emphasis is totally on empowering the patient, the therapist will tend to choose methods that serve that purpose. When therapists work at empowering, the patient is more likely to have opportunities to experience old attitudes in new contexts (Rogers, 1961a, 1961b). They have the experience of literally interacting with their therapists, of getting and giving feedback. The treatment context becomes a life-learning and life-giving context between the patient and a therapist, who responds personally and humanly. The therapist is clearly identified as a self interacting with another self. Within this context, the therapist's use of self is the main tool for change. Using self, the therapist builds trust and rapport so more risks can be taken. Use of the self by the therapist is an integral part of the therapeutic process and it should be used consciously for treatment purposes.

My Use of My Self

I have learned that, when I am fully present with the patient or family, I can move therapeutically with much greater ease. I can simultaneously reach the depths to which I need to go, and at the same time honor the fragility, the power and the sacredness of life in the other. When I am in touch with myself, my feelings, my thoughts, with what I see and hear, I am growing toward becoming a more integrated self. I am more congruent, I am more whole, and I am able to make greater contact with the other person. When I have spoken of these concepts in workshops, people thank me for speaking out, legitimizing what they have been feeling themselves. In a nutshell, what I have been describing are therapists who put their personhood and that of their patients first. It is the positive people contact that paves the way for the risks that have to be taken. Many adults have reported that they did not feel they were in contact with their parents and the others who brought them up. They did not feel like persons, but were treated as roles or expectations. If the therapeutic situation cannot bring out the people contact, then what chance does it have for really making it possible for people to feel differently themselves?

The metaphor of a musical instrument comes to mind when I think of the therapist's use of the self. How it is made, how it is cared for, its fine tuning and the ability, experience, sensitivity and creativity of the player will determine how the music will sound. Neither the player nor the instrument writes the music. A competent player with a fine instrument can play well almost any music designed for that instrument. An incompetent player with an out-of-tune instrument will vilify any music, indicating that the player has an insensitive, untrained ear. I think of the instrument as the self of the therapist: how complete one is as a person, how well one cares for oneself, how well one is tuned in to oneself, and how competent one is at one's craft. I think of the music as the presentation of the patient. How that music is heard and understood by the therapist is a large factor in determining the outcome of the therapy.

I give myself permission to be totally clear and in touch with myself. I also give myself full permission to share my views, as well as permission to see if my views have validity for the people with whom I am working. The person of the therapist is the center point around which successful therapy revolves. The theories and techniques are important. I have developed many of them. But, I see them as tools to be used in a fully human context. I further believe that therapists are responsible for the initiation and continuation of the therapy process. They are not in charge of the patients within that process.

The whole therapeutic process must be aimed at opening up the healing potential within the patient or client. Nothing really changes until that healing potential is opened. The way is through the meeting of the deepest self of the therapist with the deepest self of the person, patient or client. When this occurs, it creates a context of vulnerability, of openness to change. This clearly brings in the spiritual dimension. People already have what they need to grow; and the therapist's task is to enable patients to utilize their own resources. If I believe that human beings are sacred, then when I look at their behavior, I will attempt to help them to live up to their own sacredness. If I believe that human beings are things to be manipulated, then I will develop ways to manipulate them. If I believe that patients are victims, then I will try to rescue them. In other words, there is a close relationship between what I believe and how I act. The more in touch I am with my beliefs, and acknowledge them, the more I give myself freedom to choose how to use those beliefs.

What started as a radical idea years ago has become part of a recognized psychology, predicated upon the belief that human beings have the capacity for their own growth and healing. In this century, there has been more research and attention given to the nature of the human being than ever before. As we approach the 21st century, we know a great deal about how the body and brain work, and how we learn. We can transplant organs, we can create artificial intelligence, we can go to the moon and other planets. We can communicate anywhere in the world instantly by satellite. We can fly across the Atlantic in three hours—a trip that took several weeks a hundred years ago. We have also created the biggest monster of all time, the nuclear bomb, and we still haven't learned to accept a positive way of dealing with conflict.

Amid these changes is the growing conviction that human beings must evolve a new consciousness that places a high value on being human, that leads toward cooperation, that enables positive conflict resolution and that recognizes our spiritual foundations. Can we accept as a given that the self of the therapist is an essential factor in the therapeutic process? If this turns out to be true, it will alter our way of teaching therapists as well as treating patients.

We started out knowing that the person of the therapist could be harmful to the patient. We concentrated on ways to avoid that. Now, we need to concentrate on ways in which the use of self can be of positive value in treatment.

References

Buber, M. (1970). *I and thou.* New York: Charles Scribners.

Dreikurs, R. (1960). The current dilemma in psychotherapy. *Journal of Existential Psychology*, 1, 187.

Freud, S. (1959). *Collected papers, Volume II.* New York: Basic Books.

Hollender, M.H. Szasz, T.S. (1956). A contribution to the philosophy of medicine, *Archive of Internal Medicine.* 97, 585-592.

Jellinek, EM. (1960). *The disease concept of alcoholism.* New Haven: College and University Press.

Langs, R. (1985). *Madness and cure.* Emerson, NJ: Newconcept Press.

Maslow, A. (1962). *Toward a psychology of being.* Second Edition, New York: Van Nostrand Reinhold.

Needleman, J. (1985). *The way of the physician.* New York: Harper and Row.

Rogers, C. (1951). *Client-centered therapy.* Boston: Houghton-Mifflin.

Rogers, C. (1961a). The process equation of psychotherapy. *American Journal of Psychotherapy* 15, 27-45.

Rogers, C. (1961b). *On becoming a person.* Boston: Houghton-Mifflin.

Yalom, I. (1980). *Existential psychotherapy.* New York: Basic Books.

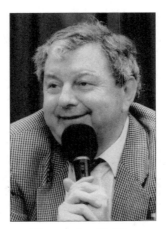

About the Editor

John Banmen, R. Psych., RMFT is internationally known as an author, therapist and educator. His training programs have taken him to over a dozen countries in Asia, Europe, South America and North America. Dr. Banmen's co-authored book, *The Satir Model: Family Therapy and Beyond* (1991), received the AAMFT/Satir Research and Education prize in 1994. He is editor of *Meditations and Inspirations* (1985) and *Meditations of Virginia Satir: Peace Within, Peace Between and Peace Among* (2003).

Dr. Banmen is the founding president of the BC Association for Marriage and Family Therapy, a former member of the Board of Directors of the American Association for Marriage and Family Therapy (AAMFT), a former member of the Board of Directors of the BC Psychological Association, a member of the Board of Directors of the International Family Therapy Association, and the Director of Training for the Satir Institute of the Pacific.

Dr. Banmen is a former honorary Associate Professor at the University of Hong Kong and was on faculty at the University of British Columbia for 21 years. He is an Approved Supervisor with AAMFT and provides extensive supervision for counselors, psychotherapists, and family therapists. He also practices privately in Delta, British Columbia, Canada, with individuals and couples in family therapy.

Two recently published books, *Application of the Satir Growth Model* (2006), and *Satir Transformational Systemic Therapy* (2007), both edited by Dr. Banmen, are soon to be published in Chinese in 2008. He is presently putting much of his time into expanding the use of the Satir Model (STST) in China.